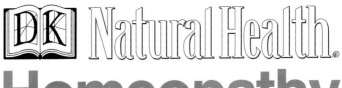

DK Natural Health®

Homeopathy
H A N D B O O K

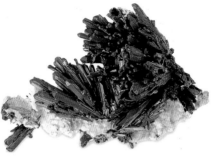

GW00372056

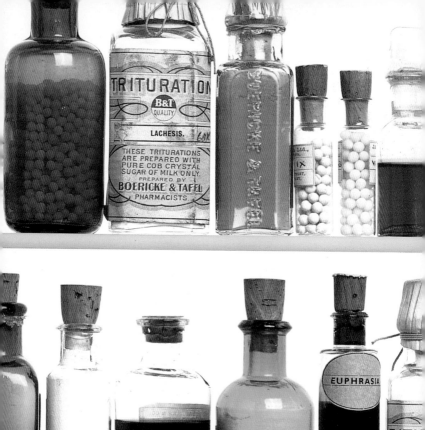

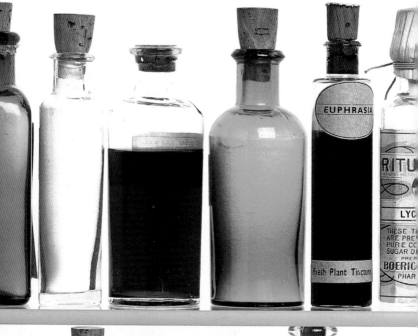

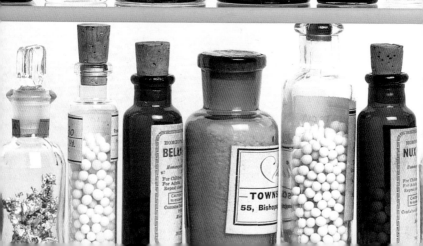

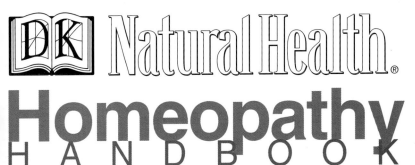

DK Natural Health®
Homeopathy
H A N D B O O K

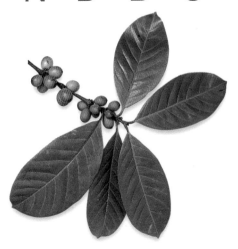

DR ANDREW LOCKIE

A Dorling Kindersley Book

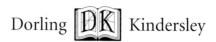

Dorling **DK** Kindersley

LONDON, NEW YORK, SYDNEY, DELHI, PARIS,
MUNICH AND JOHANNESBURG

Natural Health magazine is the leading publication inthe field of natural self-care.
For subscription information call 800-526-8440 or visit www.naturalhealthmag.com.
Natural Health® is a registered trademark of Weider Publications, Inc.

Produced for Dorling Kindersley by Walton and Pringle
www.waltonandpringle.com

Managing Editor Gillian Roberts
Managing Art Editor Tracey Ward
Category Publisher Mary-Clare Jerram
Art Director Tracy Killick
DTP Designers Louise Paddick and Louise Waller
Production Manager Maryann Webster
US Editor Crystal A. Coble
US Editorial Director LaVonne Carlson

First American Edition 2001
2 4 6 8 10 9 7 5 3 1
Published in the United States by Dorling Kindersley Publishing, Inc.,
95 Madison Avenue, New York, NY 10016

Library of Congress Cataloging-in-Publication Data

Lockie, Andrew.
    Homeopathy handbook / Andrew Lockie.
        p. cm. -- (Healing handbooks)
    "First published in Great Britain in 1999."
    Includes index.
    ISBN 0-7894-7178-7 (alk. paper)
        1. Homeopathy--Handbooks, manuals, etc. I. Title. II Series.
    RX73 .L59 2001
    615.5'.32--dc21   00-045196

Color reproduced by Colourscan, Singapore
Printed and bound in Italy by Graphicom

see our complete
catalog at
www.dk.com

Contents

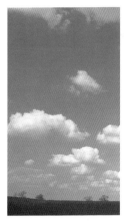 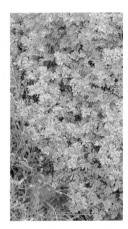 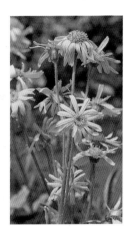

DR. ANDREW LOCKIE'S INTRODUCTION

An integrated approach to medicine can provide a flexible, pragmatic approach to healthcare; as such, homeopathy has an important role to play. By understanding the basics, you will be able to take more responsibility for your own health.

HOMEOPATHY'S ORIGINS

Medical practitioners have long looked to homeopathic-type practices to cure patients. Hippocrates and Paracelsus (*see page 10*) made discoveries that continue to affect the practice of homeopathy, but it was not until the late 18th century that a concerted breakthrough was made. It took place in Germany when Dr. Samuel Christian Hahnemann (1755–1843), disillusioned with his profession, left his career in conventional medicine to research alternative treatments. He began treating patients with a principle of "like cures like."

In 1796, Hahnemann published his first book about his new type of medicine, *A New Principle for Ascertaining the Curative Powers of Drugs and Some Examinations of Previous Principles*. He called his new system "homeopathy," from the Greek *homeo* meaning "similar" and *pathos* meaning "suffering."

UNDERSTANDING THE BASICS

The key to homeopathy is the practitioner's ability to understand and interpret a patient's symptoms – the outward signs of internal disorder – both before and after a remedy is given. Whereas in conventional medical practice, people diagnosed with the same condition will generally be given the same medicine, in homeopathy the patient is treated individually. Homeopathic practitioners take into consideration a whole host of other factors, such as temperament, state of mind, and lifestyle, before suggesting a remedy.

Homeopathy's safe, gentle approach complies with one of the most important rules of medical intervention: namely that it should do no harm. A great many common, everyday ailments may be treated safely and effectively at home with homeopathic remedies.

FOR THE LAYPERSON

My aim is to provide you with a comprehensive account of homeopathy and its uses. By understanding the basics of the practice, you can assist your body's wellbeing. There are many hundreds of homeopathic remedies available commercially, and attempting to choose the correct one can be confusing. This book aims to unravel some of the mysteries surrounding homeopathy and enable the layperson to make a more informed choice about homeopathic self-treatment.

SERIOUS AILMENTS

Under no circumstances, however, should patients suffering from serious ailments (or those uncertain of their ailment) consider self-treatment. They should always consult a recommended homeopathic practitioner or a conventional doctor.

In general, a conventional doctor should be consulted for any ailment that can be treated quickly and effectively by conventional medicine or for any condition that requires further investigation. This also applies to common ailments that worsen: a cold that develops into a chest infection, for example.

Certain serious ailments may be alleviated by homeopathy, but in the treatment of these conditions, the experience of a qualified homeopathic practitioner is essential from the outset.

COMPLEMENTARY MEDICINE

It is a truism that no one in the system of medicine can cure every illness every time in every patient. Some patients respond well to certain treatments while others, with seemingly similar symptoms, do not. In many parts of the world, conventionally trained doctors are

increasingly turning to complementary therapies, such as homeopathy, to widen the range of treatments available to them.

WHY THE CHANGE?

This response by the medical profession is, to some extent, in answer to the desires of a growing number of patients: people who wish to take more responsibility for their own health. An increasing number want to understand what they can do themselves to prevent illness and, if they do become ill, to understand the causes and determine how they can help themselves recover. Homeopathy offers a simple, effective, extremely safe, and relatively inexpensive way of accomplishing this – provided it is practiced with common sense.

SCIENTIFIC CLASSIFICATION

I have carried out much research into the scientific classifications of the substances from which homeopathic remedies are made. This was undertaken in order to correct the various errors and confusions that have crept into homeopathic medicine over the past 200 years. Incorporated into this book is the most up-to-date and scientifically accurate information available – for instance, the current biological, zoological, and mineralogical classifications have been used wherever possible. As a result, you may find that some of the Latin names used here are different from those found in earlier homeopathic textbooks.

Understanding
Homeopathy

A guide to the development of homeopathic treatment, explaining how remedies are made, how patients are assessed, how to self-assess, how to take homeopathic remedies, and how to help remedies work effectively.

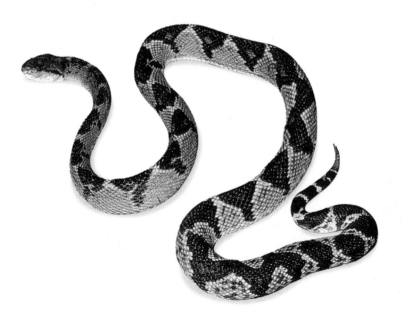

WHAT IS HOMEOPATHY?

Homeopathy is a holistic form of complementary medicine, aiming to treat the whole person, rather than just the physical symptoms. Its theories and principles date back to medicinal practices of ancient Greece and Rome.

IN THE BEGINNING

In the 5th century B.C., the Greek physician Hippocrates (460–377 B.C.) established the idea that disease resulted from natural forces rather than divine intervention, and that the patients' own powers of healing should be encouraged. At the time, medical theories were based upon the Law of Contraries, which advocated treating an illness by prescribing a substance that produced opposite or contrary symptoms to it; in contrast, Hippocrates developed the use of the Law of Similars, based on the principle that "like cures like."

PARACELSUS

For many centuries after the decline of the Roman Empire, little progress was made in the field of European medicine. Religion exerted a great influence over medical practice, and much early knowledge was forgotten.

It was when a Swiss alchemist and physician, Paracelsus (1493–1541), began to develop his theories that the study of medicine started to evolve again. He revived the ancient

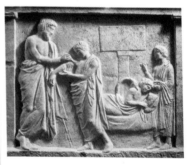

This Greek votive relief (early 4th century B.C.) illustrates ancient Greek medicinal traditions. Conventional and homeopathic medicine derive from this time.

Greek theory of the Doctrine of Signatures. This was based on the premise that the external appearance of a plant – God's "signature" – indicated the nature of its healing properties. For example, *Chelidonium majus* (greater celandine) was used to treat conditions affecting the liver and gallbladder because the yellow juice of the plant resembled bile.

Paracelsus believed disease was linked to external factors, such as contaminated food and water, rather than to mystical forces. He claimed that medical practice should be based on detailed observation and "profound knowledge of nature and her works." He believed all plants and metals contained active ingredients that could be prescribed to match specific illnesses and maintained "it depends only on the dose whether a poison is a poison or not." According to British homeopath and author James Compton Burnett (1840–1901), "Paracelsus planted the acorn from which the mighty oak of homeopathy has grown."

SAMUEL HAHNEMANN

In Germany of 1780, Dr. Samuel Hahnemann began practicing homeopathy. For nine years he worked as a conventional doctor, but grew increasingly disillusioned with the harsh medical methods of the day. He maintained that improving public hygiene, housing conditions, general health, and nutrition would do more good than the current medical practices alone.

In 1790, Hahnemann began researching a new type of medicine he called "homeopathy." He conducted tests ("provings") on himself and, later, on patients. Prior to prescription, he gave his patients a thorough physical examination and noted any existing symptoms. He questioned them closely regarding their lifestyles, general health, outlook on life, and other factors that made them feel better or worse. Following the principle of "like cures like," Hahnemann matched the patient's symptoms as closely as possible to the symptoms produced by a particular remedy and prescribed accordingly.

HAHNEMANN'S REMEDIES

In 1812 Hahnemann began teaching homeopathy at the University of Leipzig. During the course of his lifetime, he proved about 100 remedies. He also continued to develop and refine the theory and practice of the system. Despite this, the established medical world remained generally very sceptical of Hahnemann; in turn, he remained equally scornful of the established medical world.

HOMEOPATHY TODAY

By the time of Hahnemann's death (1843), homeopathy was firmly established in many parts of the world. There have been occasional periods of disenchantment, but generally its popularity continues to spread, and recent trends show a strong resurgence, particularly in the U.S. Single-remedy prescribing is prevalent worldwide, although in Germany and France the use of complex homeopathy, also known as polypharmacy (the use of combination or several remedies), is also popular. In Australia homeopathy has become strongly linked with naturopathy; while in India homeopaths have long worked successfully alongside traditional Ayurvedic medicine and conventional medicine. In the 1990s, pioneering British teachers revitalized an interest in homeopathy in Eastern Europe; in Russia it continues to be developed. In South America homeopathy has become so popular that it is taught widely in medical schools.

How Does It Work?

Homeopaths believe that good health derives from an equilibrium between the mind and body, which is maintained by a "vital force" that regulates the body's self-healing capabilities.

THE VITALISTIC CONCEPT

The vitalistic concept of science had already existed for many years by Hahnemann's time. It claims that all living things possess a subtle energy beyond their physical and chemical states, and that even inanimate matter may contain vitality. Hahnemann applied this view to both the human body and to seemingly inert substances from all the kingdoms of matter. Thus the vital force of any plant, mineral, or animal could be harnessed to produce a powerful medicine when "potentized."

Hahnemann viewed ill-health as the result of an internal imbalance affecting the body's vital force and disrupting its equilibrium. He believed that if this vital force is put under strain or weakened by this imbalance, illness may develop. In stimulating the body's self-healing abilities to fight any imbalance, Hahnemann proclaimed that the vital force produces symptoms. These may manifest themselves externally, producing such symptoms as fever or a skin rash, or may emerge as emotional or psychological states, such as weepiness or great irritability. An effective medicine must help the vital force to redress the internal imbalance, enabling the symptoms produced by that imbalance to disappear; this is what homeopaths seek to achieve.

A PERSON'S CONSTITUTION

Homeopathy works on the principle that the mind and body are so strongly linked that physical symptoms cannot be sucessfully treated without an understanding of the person's constitution and

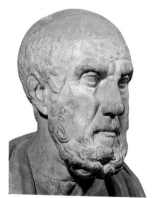

Portrait bust of Hippocrates (460–377 B.C.), known as the "father of medicine." He established the foundations of conventional and homeopathic medicine.

12

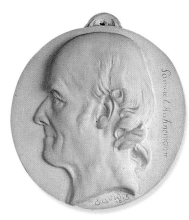

Portrait medallion of Dr. Samuel Christian Hahnemann (1755–1843). Disenchanted with conventional medicine, he began work on a new system he called "homeopathy."

character. In homeopathic terms, a person's "constitution" describes their state of health, including their temperament and any inherited and acquired characteristics. In determining constitution, a practitioner needs to ask a great many questions (*see pages 18–19*).

Homeopaths believe that healthy people resist developing sickness – despite being constantly exposed to an enormous variety of potentially harmful viruses and bacteria – as their vital force is strong and their susceptibility is therefore low.

LIKE CURES LIKE

Hahnemann developed the concept of "like cures like" (*similia similibus curentur*), first established by Hippocrates. According to this theory, substances that are capable of provoking certain symptoms in an otherwise healthy body can also act curatively on similar symptoms in a sick person. For example, *Belladonna* would be used to treat scarlet fever, since the symptoms of *Belladonna* poisoning closely resemble those of scarlet fever.

SYMPTOM PICTURES

Hahnemann's "provings" of remedies aimed to establish the particular set of symptoms – known as a "symptom picture" – produced by taking a particular substance. When the symptom picture matched the particular set of symptoms produced by an illness or imbalance in a patient, that remedy was indicated as the most effective at stimulating the vital force to treat the disorder. The key of classical homeopathy is to establish which remedy most exactly matches a patient's symptom picture.

LAWS OF CURE

As a patient progresses toward being completely cured, symptoms move from the body's inner organs (most vital) to the outer organs (less vital). Cure usually takes place from the top of the body to the bottom; as an example, head symptoms clear first, these are followed gradually by any symptoms on the extremities.

Old symptoms of illness often resurface during the homeopathic curative process, usually in the reverse order to that in which they first appeared. Immunologists claim that the body has the capacity to "remember" every "assault" on the system that it has reacted to – this process of symptoms resurfacing confirms this theory.

HOW REMEDIES ARE MADE

Homeopathic remedies are prepared to exact guidelines, but may vary in strength according to individual needs. A practitioner's skill, experience, and judgment in selecting the appropriate remedy are of paramount importance.

HAHNEMANN'S METHOD

Many of the substances from which remedies are made are highly poisonous. Hahnemann used only small amounts in his medicines, but to his consternation his patients still tended to suffer side-effects, or "aggravations" as he called them. He developed a technique called "potentization", which involved diluting the medicine and shaking it vigorously or banging it on a hard surface during preparation. This turbulent motion, which Hahnemann called "succussion", apparently released more potency into the medicine, even at lower dilutions, allowing a lower dosage to be administered.

PREPARING MATERIALS

Some plant materials may be used whole in the creation of remedies, but most raw animal and plant materials (such as leaves, roots, and flower heads) require chopping as preparation. Crystalline minerals, as well as beans or seeds, may require grinding if they are large, hard, or insoluble in water.

HOW TO MAKE TABLETS FROM ALLIUMS

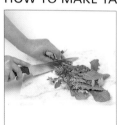

1 PREPARE RAW MATERIAL

Plant materials or animal matter must be chopped finely. Other substances can be prepared by being dissolved in water or by being ground.

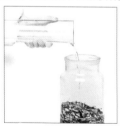

2 MIX WITH ALCOHOL

Mix the substance with alcohol and distilled water (ratios vary but 90 per cent alcohol to 10 per cent water is common). Use a large glass container for mixing.

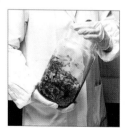

3 LEAVE TO STAND

Plant materials may stand for several weeks; mineral-based mixtures may be processed almost immediately. Longer-standing mixtures should be shaken periodically.

TRITURATION

This term describes the process of changing insoluble metals into powder. Metals that are insoluble in their natural states are combined with lactose sugar crystals; they are then ground repeatedly until they form a powder that is fine enough to be soluble in water.

COMBINING INGREDIENTS

When the raw ingredients have been prepared, they are mixed with a solution of alcohol and distilled water. The ratio of this solution varies according to the substance with which it is being mixed. The mixture is then left to stand for anything from a few moments to several weeks. This stage is known as "maceration". Mineral-based mixtures may be moved on to the next stage almost at once, whereas certain plant-based mixtures may need weeks. Those that are left to stand for a while may require occasional shaking.

THE MOTHER TINCTURE

Liquid is extracted from the mixture (either by straining or pressing) to produce what is known as the "mother tincture". This is then added to a second solution of pure alcohol and distilled water, made up according to one of several scales. The most commonly used are the decimal scale (in which the dilution factor is 1:10) and the centesimal scale (in which the dilution factor is 1:100). The tincture is succussed and diluted as many times as is necessary to achieve the required potency for the homeopathic remedy.

EXERCISE CAUTION

This information is not intended as a guide to making remedies. Unlike herbal remedies, homeopathic remedies should never be made in the home; they are prepared under strict conditions by a commercial manufacturer and should be obtained from a reputable supplier.

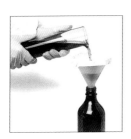

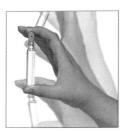

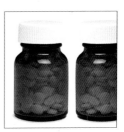

4 STRAIN THE LIQUID
When it is ready, strain the mixture through a filter or push it through a press to extract the liquid. This is the "mother tincture"; it should be stored in a dark glass jar.

5 SUCCUSS THE MIXTURE
To succuss the liquid, shake it vigorously or bang the jar firmly on a hard surface. Hahnemann coined the term "succussion"; he believed it "potentized" the liquid.

6 IMPREGNATE TABLETS
When the tincture is the correct strength and potency, add the required amount of drops to lactose tablets, granules, or powder. Store in dark glass bottles.

REMEDY STRENGTHS

Remedies are prepared to exact guidelines, but vary in strength according to the patient's needs. The practitioner's skill, experience, and judgment are responsible for selecting the appropriate remedy and its strength.

HAHNEMANN'S RULES

Hahnemann wrote precise guidelines in which methods and measurements were all strictly and scientifically controlled. He developed a unique process called "potentization," which allowed the full strength, or potency, of the substance to be released into the remedy mixture.

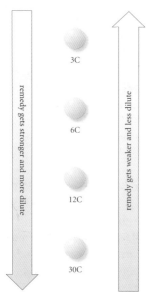

The more dilute a remedy, the stronger it is, and the higher the number or "potency"; a less dilute remedy is not as strong and has a lower number ("potency").

DILUTION

As many remedies are based on extremely poisonous or highly active ingredients, they needed to be diluted to eliminate the risk of patients suffering adverse effects. Because they are diluted to such a great degree, it is highly unlikely that even a single molecule of the original substance remains. This means that, although remedies may be based on highly poisonous substances, they are completely safe to use, even on children.

THE NUMBERING SYSTEM

Hahnemann made a surprising discovery: the more dilute the remedy, the fewer doses are needed. More dilute remedies are therefore stronger, producing a longer action and deeper effect than less dilute remedies. When recording his works, Hahnemann gave stronger remedies high numbers, denoting their higher potency, and vice versa.

Remedies usually have a number, such as *6c* or *12x*, after the name. This number indicates how many times a remedy has been diluted and succussed, and on which scale

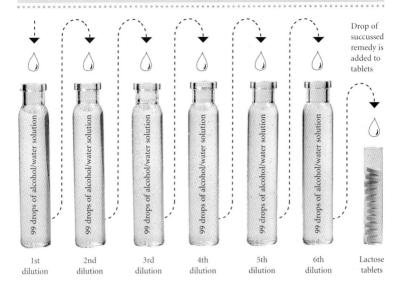

Drop of succussed remedy is added to tablets

| 1st dilution | 2nd dilution | 3rd dilution | 4th dilution | 5th dilution | 6th dilution | Lactose tablets |

(99 drops of alcohol/water solution)

(*see above*). For example, the remedy *Allium cepa 6c* has been diluted and succussed six times on the centesimal scale.

SCALES OF DILUTION

Homeopathic remedies are generally prepared according to one of two scales: the decimal (*x*) and the centesimal (*c*) (*see page 15*). More rarely, however, scales such as the millesimal (*m*) and quinquagintamillesimal (*lm*) are prepared. According to these scales, remedies are diluted by factors of 1:1,000 and 1:50,000 respectively. The millesimal is advocated mainly when a single, high-potency dose of a remedy is required; the quinquagintamillesimal is used for stubborn, chronic cases that seem to require the prescription of a "megadose" of a particular remedy.

PREPARING A POTENCY

The mother tincture (*see page 15*) is usually diluted in a mixture (the

The mother tincture is usually diluted with a mixture of alcohol and water; it is then succussed. This is repeated as many times as necessary to produce the required potency.

ratio of which varies) made from pure alcohol and distilled water, according to one of the scales. To produce a 1c potency, one drop of the mother tincture is added to 99 drops of an alcohol-and-water mixture and succussed. To produce a 2c potency, one drop of the 1c mixture is added to 99 drops of alcohol and water and succussed. This is repeated until the required potency results.

CHOOSING THE POTENCY

The potency prescribed is gauged by the homeopath according to several factors, such as the condition to be treated, the strength of the patient, and the circumstances. Not only must the remedy given be suitable, but the potency chosen must also be appropriate to the individual patient.

HOW PATIENTS ARE ASSESSED

As the basis of homeopathic assessment, a practitioner collects a wealth of information about a patient, to build up an overview of the symptoms. The charts below show the type of information a homeopath will require.

BODY

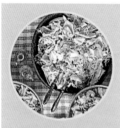

Diet plays an important role in physical wellbeing

PHYSICAL WELLBEING
- General symptoms and ailments.
- Weight, shape, and physical condition.
- Diet: food preferences and aversions, food intolerances, deficiencies, any special requirements.
- Energy levels.
- Sleep: amount, quality, dreams.
- Risks to health: smoking, alcohol consumption, recreational drugs, dangerous jobs and pastimes.
- Time out: relaxation methods, leisure activities.
- Knowledge of what to do if ill or injured.

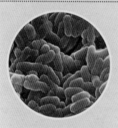

A homeopath needs to know your medical history

MEDICAL HISTORY
- Personal medical history and history of treatments.
- Family medical history: incidence in family of conditions such as heart disease, diabetes, mental health problems, or cancer.
- Inherited susceptibilities, such as allergies.
- Diet: food intolerances, susceptibility to obesity.
- Awareness of symptoms of genetically inherited disease and preventative measures.
- Checkups: self-examination, regular medical tests or screening.

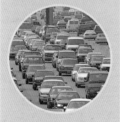

Knowing about a patient's environment is vital

ENVIRONMENT
- Climate: effects of seasonal changes and day-to-day weather patterns.
- Access to and appreciation of fresh air.
- Exposure to sun and awareness of risks.
- Effects of pollution: air, water, noise.
- Work environment: location, amount of space.
- Home environment: allergies to household products, toiletries, animals, tobacco smoke.
- Daily routine: stress and other effects of commuting, working long hours.

THE INDIVIDUAL PATIENT

◆ **THE PERSON AS PRODUCT**
Homeopaths regard a person as the product of their physical and mental wellbeing or ill-health, genetic make-up, and daily experience.

◆ **PROFILING PATIENTS**
A person's symptoms are seen as reliable clues to the most suitable remedy to activate the self-healing powers of the individual's "vital force." Characteristics of bodily functions and functional disturbances are also noted.

ADAPTATIONS

An individual's unique adaptations to their surroundings and their idiosyncratic ways are accepted and respected for making an individual what they are. The way they adapt to new home, family, or work environments; their reactions to external circumstances; their past and present experiences; and their general state of mind are all key attributes of patient assessment.

MIND

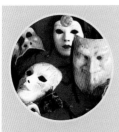

Everyone responds to events in different ways

PERSONALITY
- Temperament: relaxed, nervous, passive, assertive.
- Self-image and self-worth.
- Emotions: positive, negative, expression of, control.
- Relationships: sex drive, ability to resolve conflict, sensitivity to others, desire for approval.
- Fears, any feelings of guilt, insecurity, degree of control over personal destiny.
- Ability to cope under stress.
- Opportunities for personal expression.
- Spirituality, deeply held beliefs, motivation.

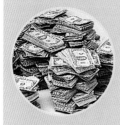

Events that happen early in life can have later effects

LIFE EVENTS
- Childhood trauma: death or other loss, abuse.
- Family circumstances: births, marriages, separations, divorce, death, children leaving home, caring for elderly or disabled relatives.
- Proximity of family and friends.
- Ability to deal with serious health problems.
- Property: buying, moving, serious alterations.
- Work experience: new job, loss of job, redundancy, relocation, overwork, juggling work and family.
- Financial or legal problems.

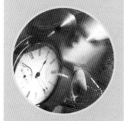

These points are crucial to creating symptom pictures

LIFE MANAGEMENT
- Time management, ability to: set realistic goals, plan and organize, cope with deadlines, delegate tasks.
- Ability to maintain a successful balance: between work and play, work and family.
- Stress management: opportunities to relax, control of stressful situations, turning problems around.
- Work: environment, physical stresses, workload.
- Routines that have been developed in order to give structure to the working day and home.
- Financial planning and organization.

HOW TO SELF-ASSESS

Homeopathic remedies can be used effectively and safely by lay people to treat many minor ailments and injuries. Careful observation enables a person to select a remedy to match their own symptoms.

SELF-PRESCRIPTION

Before starting homeopathic treatment, you must first decide whether or not it is safe to self-prescribe. Some symptoms may be indicative of a serious ailment and require the immediate attention of a conventional doctor. If pharmaceutical drugs are already being taken, it may be necessary to consult a doctor before considering extra medication. Babies, small children, pregnant women, the elderly, and those with chronic medical conditions need extra careful consideration.

IDENTIFYING SYMPTOMS

A diagnostic picture needs to be compiled in order to self-prescribe. A homeopathic practitioner would ask a person to describe themselves in terms of basic temperament, moods, feelings, and beliefs. This includes temporary psychological factors associated with their symptoms, such as irritability or an aversion to sympathy. Also of significance are details about any emotional traumas – from deep-seated childhood experiences to events of the recent past, such as bereavement. Details of how the weather, seasons, and times of day affect the individual, personal likes and dislikes, and in particular objects of fear, are all important in helping to build up a complex picture.

ASSESSING LIFESTYLE

When assessing yourself, general features of your lifestyle should be taken into consideration. Dietary factors of significance include caffeine, alcohol, and tobacco consumption, food preferences and aversions, and potential sources of irritation or digestive upset. Stress levels are also significant. You should look carefully at how much stress is caused by work, at the amount of time you have for relaxation and for following interests, whether you get enough sleep, and the amount, and type, of exercise you take.

SYMPTOM PICTURES

A "symptom picture" is compiled from all the information provided by a patient, making use of external information as well as the bodily ailments. Make a note of the characteristics of the symptoms suffered or noticed (if prescribing for someone else, also make a note of what you can see and everything they tell you). Some symptoms may be associated with other ailments or with a particular state of mind and it is necessary to ascertain all such information before deciding on a course of action. Armed with a symptom picture, a person can look at the charts and remedies profiled in this book and identify suitable treatment. It should be noted that it is not necessary to exhibit all the symptoms listed in order for a particular remedy to be suitable. The remedy can be chosen on the basis of the main symptoms, the likely cause, and the characteristics of their onset.

SAFETY ISSUES

There are several rules to remember before self-prescribing.

• Consult a conventional doctor for serious or unknown ailments, or if there is no improvement in two to three weeks (48 hours in children under five).

• Do not stop taking any prescribed conventional medicine without first consulting a conventional doctor.

• Tell your doctor about any homeopathic remedies you take.

DIAGNOSTIC CHECKLIST

QUESTIONS	EXAMPLE ANSWERS
WHAT ARE YOUR MOST OBVIOUS PHYSICAL SYMPTOMS?	Pain, soreness, inflammation, skin eruption, itching, bleeding, nausea, vomiting, diarrhea, sore throat, cough, fever, fainting, dizziness, headache.
ARE MAIN SYMPTOMS ACCOMPANIED BY LESS ACUTE SYMPTOMS?	Perspiration, chilliness, great thirst, desire for or aversion to certain foods, loss of appetite, sensitivity to touch, weak limbs, coated tongue, swollen glands.
WHAT ARE THE CHAR-ACTERISTICS OF YOUR SYMPTOMS?	Location in the body, sudden or gradual onset, constant or intermittent occurrence, frequency, or recurrence.
DO YOU HAVE ANY PSYCHOLOGICAL SYMPTOMS?	Restlessness, irritability, anger, anxiety, tearfulness, self-pity, emotional oversensitivity, indifference, desire to be alone, irrational fears, desire for sympathy.
ARE YOU AWARE OF ANY OBVIOUS CAUSE OF YOUR SYMPTOMS?	Injury, viral infection, bacterial infection, exposure to extremes of temperature or strong wind, stress, anxiety, grief, overwork.
DO YOUR SYMPTOMS IMPROVE OR WORSEN IN CERTAIN CONDITIONS?	Warmth or cold, fresh air, application of hot or cold compresses, sitting or standing, lying in a particular way, physical or mental exertion, emotional stress.

HOW TO TAKE REMEDIES

Homeopathic remedies come in several different forms; the choice of which type to use depends upon personal preference as well as upon the patient's aptitude for taking medication.

TYPES OF REMEDIES

Lactose tablets are the most common form of homeopathic remedy, although sucrose tablets are available for those who suffer from lactose-intolerance. Because these tablets can be dissolved under the tongue, a remedy is able to enter the bloodstream directly.

Remedies are also available as pilules, granules, or powder, and mother tinctures may be diluted to make soothing solutions, or used in the creation of ointments and creams. The latter can be applied directly onto the skin. You may also see remedies sold as "biochemic tissue salts." These are minerals that can be taken alone or as part of a combination with other homeopathic remedies to treat common ailments.

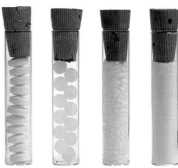

Different forms of homeopathic remedy, shown from left to right: tablets, pilules, granules, and powder.

INDIVIDUAL NEEDS

Given the highly individualistic nature of homeopathic prescription, two people are unlikely to be prescribed the same remedy, even if their symptoms appear to be identical. For the same reason, patients may find that their remedies do not match any of the general profiles of remedies listed for their ailment in popular homeopathic course books.

One remedy may be prescribed constitutionally to address the underlying causes of an ailment, for instance bodily imbalances, with another remedy prescribed for a specific, acute symptom. Also, one remedy may be substituted for another on a subsequent visit to the practitioner, depending on the patient's progress.

PROMOTING RECOVERY

Unless a qualified practitioner has recommended a combination of homeopathic remedies (*see left*) it is best to take only one at a time. One reason for this is that a remedy's effectiveness may be lessened if used in combination. Taking remedies individually also allows for assessment of the efficacy of the remedy: the decision to repeat the dosage (or the remedy itself) relies on the practitioner's being able to discover whether or not a remedy has worked by figuring out whether the symptoms have improved.

All homeopathic remedies work best when combined with good nutrition, exercise, a low-stress environment, and emotional and intellectual states that promote a balanced body system.

FOLLOWING THE RULES

In order to take homeopathic remedies effectively, it is important to follow the rules for maximizing effects (*see right*). The reasons for doing so are are as follows:

• Patients should try to leave at least 30 minutes after eating before taking a remedy so it enters the system by itself.

• Likewise it is important not to eat for 30 minutes after taking a remedy so as not to inhibit absorption.

• The recommendation to avoid strong foods and drinks is due to the fact that they may affect the body's system – some, such as coffee, may actually counteract the remedy.

• Strong household cleaners and other such chemical products may actually have a poisoning effect on the body.

• Avoiding certain medical substances is important because they may inhibit a remedy from working on its own. If in doubt, consult your practitioner.

• Avoid touching homeopathic remedies; this can prevent them from working effectively. Remedies should be taken with a clean, dry spoon, or dropped into the mouth, without being touched by the fingers. If tablets are touched or dropped, they should not be returned to the container.

• When storing homeopathic remedies, make sure the tops are securely in place. Also make sure they are kept in a suitable location and temperature.

MAXIMIZING EFFECTS

When taking a homeopathic remedy, observe the following "rules" to make sure it has the best chance of working effectively.

• Do not eat for 30 mins before taking a remedy.

• Do not eat for 30 mins after taking a remedy.

• Avoid strong foods and drinks, such as spicy foods and alcohol or consume them only in moderation.

• Avoid brushing your teeth 30 mins before or after taking a remedy.

• Avoid using strong substances, such as household cleaning products.

• Avoid medicinal substances and certain products such as some essential oils such as eucalyptus and peppermint.

• Do not touch or handle a remedy.

• Store homeopathic products properly.

HELPING REMEDIES TO WORK

A homeopathic remedy helps the body heal itself.
This self-healing can be encouraged, and future health
and well-being promoted, by a series of measures
put into place alongside the treatment.

COMPLEMENTARY LIFESTYLE GUIDE

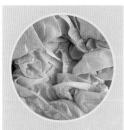

Eating regular meals is important for good health

EATING FOR HEALTH

- Eat vegetarian proteins rather than meat and dairy.
- Eat foods rich in minerals and vitamins, or take supplements.
- Cut down on refined carbohydrates, salt, processed foods, sugar, animal fats, yeast, caffeine, and alcohol.
- Drink plenty of fluids.
- Lose weight if necessary.
- Consult a dietician about specific needs.
- Include plenty of fiber in the diet.
- Cook healthily: for instance, broil instead of fry.

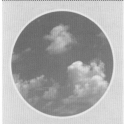

Strong household products are potential irritants

IMPROVING SURROUNDINGS

- Prohibit smoking at home and at work.
- Reduce allergies by keeping the home dust-free.
- Use environmentally friendly household products.
- Avoid perfumed toiletries and skincare products.
- Avoid polluted or noisy environments.
- Humidify or dehumidify rooms as necessary.
- Make sure rooms are draft-free but have adequate ventilation.
- Wear natural fibers.
- Create an area that is conducive to relaxation.

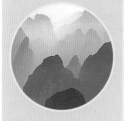

Spending time in natural settings can relieve stress

MANAGING STRESS

- Take periods of rest during the day and get enough sleep at night.
- Make time for relaxation and exercise each day.
- Prioritize and organize tasks.
- Delegate and learn to say "no" to extra work.
- Eat properly and regularly; get plenty of fresh air.
- Make time for leisure activities and socializing.
- Take a vacation.
- Cultivate a positive attitude to all things.
- Face up to problems rather than putting them off.

PROMOTING GOOD HEALTH

◆ **SELF-HEALING**

While not necessarily providing an instant cure, a homepathic remedy is believed to encourage the body's self-healing mechanisms and to nurture a sense of wellbeing, good energy levels, and a resistance to ill-health.

◆ **A SENSE OF WELLBEING**

In order to heal physical symptoms, it is important to take a look at the mind. A positive mental attitude is a crucial tool in getting better physically.

THE HOLISTIC VIEW

All homeopathic remedies can be helped to work by adopting a lifestyle that will promote good health and a positive outlook. Eating a balanced diet and getting regular exercise are of obvious benefit; however, homeopaths also need to look at other aspects of a person's life – such as their outlook on life and external circumstances – before deciding on treatment.

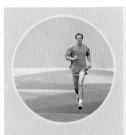

Warm up and cool down before and after exercise

KEEPING FIT

- Learn breathing techniques to maximize the benefits of exercise.
- Include exercise in a daily routine.
- Plan a weekly exercise program.
- Aim to improve your energy levels, brain-power, and mood.
- Choose activities for specific purposes, such as muscle coordination, strength, or endurance.
- Use exercise as a means of getting time to yourself, or meeting people, or as a challenge.

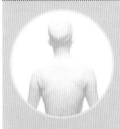

Manipulation can ease spine and joint disorders

TREATMENTS FOR THE BODY

- Breathing and relaxation techniques: for relief of pain and stress-related symptoms.
- Touch therapies: pressure or massage for general wellbeing and health (aromatherapy, reflexology).
- Manipulation: for bone and muscle disorders, and body alignment (physiotherapy, osteopathy).
- Physical re-education: for tension release, posture, and flexibility (Pilates, Alexander technique).
- Movement therapies: for increased vitality and self-healing (t'ai chi, yoga, dance movement therapy).

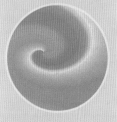

Hypnotherapy can be used to desensitize pain

TREATMENTS FOR THE MIND

- Breathing and relaxation techniques: for managing stress and treating mental conditions.
- Meditation: focusing on feelings of inner peace and fulfillment rather than on thought processes.
- Psychotherapy and counseling: talking to a skilled listener treats mental and emotional disorders.
- Hypnotherapy: using a trancelike, conscious state to influence physical and mental conditions.
- Creative therapies: use of sounds, music, or art to treat mental and emotional disorders.

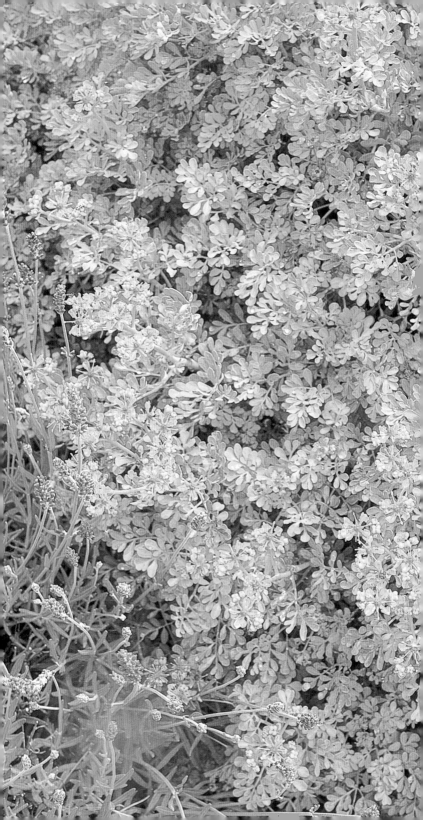

Choosing
a Remedy

A visual guide to 72 key homeopathic remedies

with details of their actions and current uses.

Also included are key homeopathic preparations

and practical self-help advice.

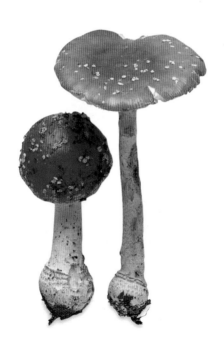

ARSEN. ALB.

Key remedy for asthma and breathlessness

Calms digestive disorders ◆ Treats skin complaints

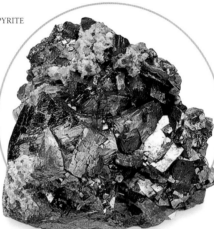

ARSENOPYRITE forms as prismatic crystals.

Crystals have a metallic luster and when heated or struck, they give off a smell of garlic.

This mineral is the main ore of arsenic.

Arsenopyrite is found in Sweden, Germany, Norway, England, and Canada.

KEY ACTIONS

- AIDS WITH BREATHING
- TREATS VOMITING AND DIARRHEA
- EASES HEADACHES
- HEALS SKIN PROBLEMS

KEY PREPARATIONS

- TINCTURE Arsenic is triturated by being ground repeatedly with lactose sugar until it is soluble in water. It is then diluted and succussed.

INDICATIONS

● **RESPIRATORY ILLNESS**
Arsen. alb. is a key remedy used for asthma and breathlessness. It is given chiefly to treat disorders of the mucous membranes of the respiratory and digestive tracts.

● **DIGESTIVE DISORDERS**
It is prescribed for violent digestive upsets with diarrhea and vomiting, such as gastroenteritis and colitis. These are often aggravated by stress and anxiety, and may be accompanied by fever.

● **CANDIDIASIS**
Arsen. alb. is prescribed for the treatment of

Candidiasis (yeast infection), which is characterized by a burning, offensive-smelling discharge and inflammation of the genitals.

● **HEADACHES**
Arsen. alb. is used for easing the pain of headaches and associated vomiting and nausea.

● **ANXIETY**
Effective for treating physical and mental anxiety.

● **CAUTION**
In the past, doctors of conventional medicine used arsenic to treat eczema, but it is now considered too toxic.

NITRIC AC.

Calms painful skin ailments ◆ Eases rhinitis

Used to treat warts, hemorrhoids, and anal fissures

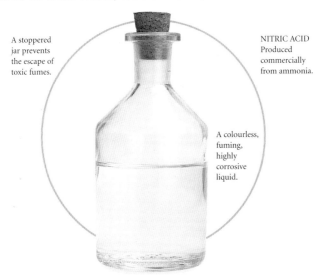

A stoppered jar prevents the escape of toxic fumes.

NITRIC ACID Produced commercially from ammonia.

A colourless, fuming, highly corrosive liquid.

KEY ACTIONS

- RELIEVES RHINITIS
- TREATS MOUTH ULCERS
- HELPS RELIEVE HEMORRHOIDS AND ANAL FISSURES
- HELPS CURE WARTS

KEY PREPARATIONS

- TINCTURE made by diluting one part nitric acid in nine parts alcohol. This mixture is then diluted and succussed.

INDICATIONS

● **CANCER**
Nitric acid is associated with treatment for cancer of the breast, stomach, uterus, and glands in the later stages.

● **SKIN AILMENTS**
Painful skin ailments, especially where the mucous membranes meet the skin of the mouth, nose, or anus, are treated with *Nitric acid*. It is also used to treat warts, anal fissures, hemorrhoids, and mouth ulcers.

● **RHINITIS**
Rhinitis is characterized by pain in the nostrils and possible nosebleeds. It is worsened by cold, damp air, and the consumption of fatty foods and milk. *Nitric acid* is used to alleviate the symptoms.

● **CANDIDIASIS**
Candidiasis affects males and females. It is a fungus that lives in warm, moist conditions, thriving if the immune system is low. *Nitric acid* is used to treat candidiasis as well as blisters and ulcers on the genitals.

● **CAUTION**
Nitric acid is produced from ammonia. This acid is highly corrosive and gives off fumes that are extremely irritant and toxic if inhaled. The acid should be kept in a stoppered jar.

PHOSPHORIC AC.

Calms exam nerves ◆ Assists conventional medicine

used by diabetics ◆ Relieves headaches

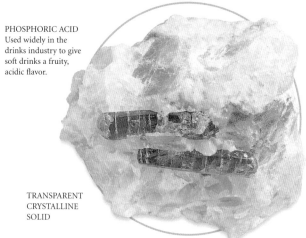

PHOSPHORIC ACID
Used widely in the
drinks industry to give
soft drinks a fruity,
acidic flavor.

Phosphoric acid
is dissolved in
alcohol to make
the remedy.

TRANSPARENT
CRYSTALLINE
SOLID

KEY ACTIONS

- ALLEVIATES INSOMNIA
- RELIEVES MILD DIARRHEA
- EASES GROWING PAINS
- TREATS EXHAUSTION

KEY PREPARATIONS

- TINCTURE *Phosphoric acid* is dissolved in alcohol in a ratio of 1:9. It is then repeatedly diluted and succussed.

INDICATIONS

● **GRIEF**
Phosphoric acid is used in the treatment of grief associated with great exhaustion.

● **DIABETES**
Homeopathic treatment for diabetes is recommended in support of conventional medicine. Prescription depends upon the symptoms, but *Phosphoric acid* is effective when emotional stress has played a part in the onset of diabetes.

● **CFS**
Phosphoric acid is prescribed for weakness in the spinal cord and associated nerves, which are often symptoms of Chronic Fatigue Syndrome (CFS). The condition is also known as ME (myalgic encephalomyelitis), or post-viral syndrome.

● **MILD DIARRHEA**
Travelers should consider taking *Phosphoric acid* in their first aid kit, as it is effective in treating mild cases of diarrhea.

● **CAUTION**
Homeopathic medicine can assist with grieving. Treatment of long-term depression, however, may require psychiatric help, in conjunction with antidepressant drugs, psychotherapy, and counseling.

ACONITE

Eases childhood sleeplessness ◆ Soothes sore th

dry, irritating coughs ◆ Helps with emotional pro...ms

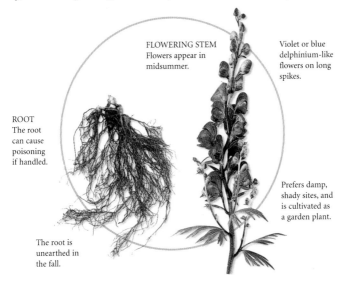

FLOWERING STEM
Flowers appear in
midsummer.

Violet or blue
delphinium-like
flowers on long
spikes.

ROOT
The root
can cause
poisoning
if handled.

Prefers damp,
shady sites, and
is cultivated as
a garden plant.

The root is
unearthed in
the fall.

KEY ACTIONS

- SOOTHING
- EMOTIONALLY CALMING
- EASES DIFFICULT
  RESPIRATION
- RELIEVES HEADACHES

KEY PREPARATIONS

- TINCTURE which is
  made from the
  whole plant, which is
  unearthed during
  the flowering season,
  chopped, and
  macerated in alcohol.

INDICATIONS

● **FEVER**
A sudden rise in
temperature, particularly
when accompanied by an
inflamed throat or a dry,
irritating cough, can be
alleviated by *Aconite*.
Dosage varies according
to the symptoms.

● **BRONCHITIS**
Aconite is prescribed to
treat bronchitis that
comes on suddenly after
exposure to cold, dry air.

● **CHILDBIRTH**
Used to relieve a strong
fear of impending death
experienced by a mother
during labor. Also treats
urine retention in either
the mother or baby.

● **SLEEPLESSNESS**
Poor sleeping patterns in
infants or children can be
caused by a variety of
factors. *Aconite* can help
calm a child worried by
an inability to sleep or
frightened by nightmares.

● **PHOBIAS AND FEARS**
Aconite is used to treat
several anxiety states.
Particularly for patients
who have a fear of dying.

● **HEADACHES**
Pulsating headaches that
come on suddenly can be
relieved by *Aconite*.

● **CAUTION**
**High doses of *Aconite*
should not be taken
internally due to its
toxic nature.**

AGARICUS

Used to treat palpitations ◆ Assists alongside conventional medicine for Multiple Sclerosis ◆ Calms anxiety

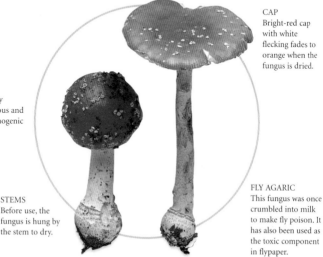

CAP
Bright-red cap with white flecking fades to orange when the fungus is dried.

A highly poisonous and hallucinogenic fungus.

STEMS
Before use, the fungus is hung by the stem to dry.

FLY AGARIC
This fungus was once crumbled into milk to make fly poison. It has also been used as the toxic component in flypaper.

KEY ACTIONS

- USED TO ASSIST SUFFERERS OF PARKINSON'S DISEASE
- CALMING
- ASSISTS WITH HEART IRREGULARITIES
- SOOTHES CHILBLAINS

KEY PREPARATIONS

- TINCTURE made from the Fly Agaric toadstool. The whole, fresh fungus may be used, or the dried cap. It is washed thoroughly and ground into a mash before being steeped in alcohol. It is then strained, diluted, and succussed.

INDICATIONS

● **MUSCLE SPASMS**
These can be indicative of Parkinson's Disease (characterized by general weakness and trembling limbs among other symptoms) or Multiple Sclerosis (characterized by weak, shaky movements accompanied by shooting pains). *Agaricus* may be prescribed to assist conventional medicine.

● **PALPITATIONS**
Palpitations occur for many reasons; *Agaricus* is associated with those induced by stimulants.

● **CHILBLAINS**
Chilblains are common on the hands and feet.

They can be treated effectively with *Agaricus*.

● **TWITCHING EYELIDS**
Agaricus is prescribed for eyelid twitching when there is no other bodily twitching, indicating tiredness or anxiety.

● **CAUTION**
The Fly Agaric toadstool, from which *Agaricus* derives, has been used for centuries in traditional and shamanic medicine. However, it is highly toxic if taken without preparation. A severe overdose can be fatal, while a mild overdose can cause nausea, vomiting, diarrhea, breathing problems, and confusion.

ALLIUM CEPA

Eases neuralgia ◆ Treats cold and influenza

Alleviates allergies, including hay fever

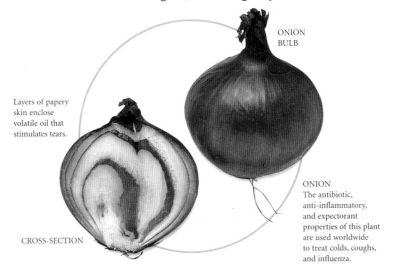

ONION
BULB

Layers of papery
skin enclose
volatile oil that
stimulates tears.

ONION
The antibiotic,
anti-inflammatory,
and expectorant
properties of this plant
are used worldwide
to treat colds, coughs,
and influenza.

CROSS-SECTION

KEY ACTIONS

- EASES RHINITIS
- FIGHTS INFECTION
- SOOTHES IRRITATED EYES

KEY PREPARATIONS

- TINCTURE made from the mature bulb, gathered in summer. It is steeped in alcohol before being filtered, diluted, and succussed.
- POULTICE used in traditional medicine for the treatment of chilblains, infections, and arthritis.
- EATEN to thin and purify the blood and as an aid to clearing gastric and bronchial infections.

INDICATIONS

● **NEURALGIA**
Allium cepa is used to treat burning neuralgic pain that alternates from one side of the body to the other.

● **COLDS & INFECTION**
Onion causes the eyes and nose to water, and is used homeopathically to treat conditions that cause the same reaction in the body, such as influenza and colds. Antibiotic and antiseptic, it is also used to fight other forms of infection, such as of the chest or throat.

● **HAY FEVER**
Acute symptoms of hay fever, especially those accompanied by profuse watering of the eyes and irritating, burning mucus, can be treated with *Allium cepa*. To be fully effective, it may need to be taken in conjunction with several other homeopathic remedies.

● **RHINITIS**
Allium cepa eases the symptoms of watery mucus that burns the skin of the nose and the upper lip, causing it to become painful.

● **POSTOPERATIVE**
After amputation, many patients suffer from what is known as "phantom limb pain"; *Allium cepa* may be used as a pain-relieving treatment.

ALOE

Soothes grazes, scalds, and sunburn ◆ Calms varicose veins

Helps Irritable Bowel Syndrome and constipation

The gel of this plant, found in the leaves, has a long history of medicinal uses as a skin lotion.

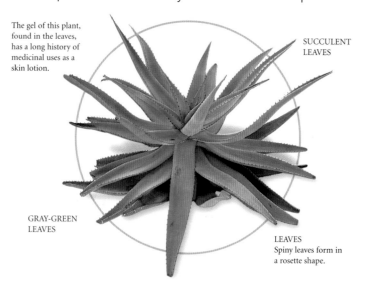

SUCCULENT LEAVES

GRAY-GREEN LEAVES

LEAVES
Spiny leaves form in a rosette shape.

KEY ACTIONS

- HEALS WOUNDS
- EMOLLIENT
- STIMULATES SECRETION OF BILE
- LAXATIVE

KEY PREPARATIONS

- BITTER ALOES The leaves exude a bitter liquid which is dried and known as "bitter aloes." This is used by herbalists to treat constipation.
- GEL Leaves are broken off and the clear gel is applied to the skin as a first aid remedy for burns.
- TINCTURE made from bitter aloes. Used to stimulate the appetite.

INDICATIONS

● **BEAUTY TREATMENT**
Aloe has a long history as a skin lotion – Cleopatra is said to have attributed her beauty to it.

● **FIRST AID**
Aloe is an excellent first aid remedy to keep in the home for burns, grazes, scalds, and sunburn. A leaf, broken off, releases soothing gel, which may be applied to the affected part.

● **LAXATIVE**
The bitter yellow liquid in the leaves (bitter aloes) are stongly laxative. They cause the colon to contract, generally producing a bowel

movement 8–12 hours after consumption.

● **SKIN CONDITIONS**
The gel is useful for skin conditions that need soothing and astringing, and will help varicose veins to some degree.

● **ULCERS**
The protective and healing effect of *Aloe* also works internally, and the gel can be used for peptic ulcers and irritable bowel syndrome.

● **CAUTION**
Do not use bitter aloes on the skin. Do not take during pregnancy. Do not take if suffering from hemorrhoids or kidney disease.

ALUMINA

Treats senile dementia and Alzheimer's disease

Alleviates fatigue ◆ Relieves constipation

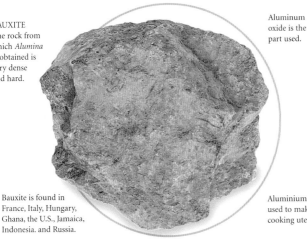

BAUXITE
The rock from which *Alumina* is obtained is very dense and hard.

Aluminum oxide is the part used.

Bauxite is found in France, Italy, Hungary, Ghana, the U.S., Jamaica, Indonesia. and Russia.

Aluminium is also used to make cooking utensils.

KEY ACTIONS

- STIMULATES SLUGGISH BOWELS
- TREATS CONFUSION AND FAILING MEMORY
- EMOTIONALLY CALMING

KEY PREPARATIONS

- CRYSTALS of aluminum oxide are extracted from bauxite using an industrial process. They are then triturated with lactose sugar, filtered, diluted, and succussed.

INDICATIONS

● **DEMENTIA**
Alumina may be prescribed to help stem the alleviation of mental processes leading to sluggish and absent-minded behavior, often associated with senile dementia and Alzheimer's disease. Elderly people are most commonly affected.

● **DIGESTION**
Traditionally used as an antacid in indigestion remedies, *Alumina* can also be found in food additives, baking powder, and drinking water.

● **CONSTIPATION**
There are different types of constipation; *Alumina* may be prescribed when a patient experiences difficulty with passing even soft stools.

● **NERVOUS DISORDERS**
Alumina is given to treat nervous complaints, particularly those characterized by a sense of muscle paralysis and fatigue. It may also be prescribed for delicate babies.

● **CAUTION**
Significant amounts of *Alumina* absorbed into the body are thought by some to cause the mental processes to slow down. Some evidence suggests that it may aid the development of Alzheimer's disease.

ANACARDIUM OCC.

Helps with exam nerves ◆ Soothes irritated skin

Effectively treats certain forms of depression

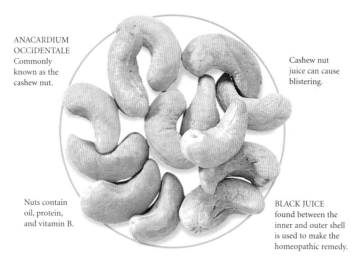

ANACARDIUM OCCIDENTALE Commonly known as the cashew nut.

Cashew nut juice can cause blistering.

Nuts contain oil, protein, and vitamin B.

BLACK JUICE found between the inner and outer shell is used to make the homeopathic remedy.

KEY ACTIONS

- REDUCES STRESS
- RELIEVES ANXIETY
- SOOTHING
- RELIEVES DEPRESSION

KEY PREPARATIONS

- TINCTURE made from the black juice found between the outer and inner shell of the cashew nut. It is dissolved in alcohol, then diluted and succussed.

INDICATIONS

● **EXAM NERVES**
Anacardium occ. is prescribed for extreme cases of anxiety about taking exams. It assists with the student's feeling of inability to remember important information. The treatment should be taken regularly before an exam. The remedy may be effective when prescribed for performers suffering from stage fright.

● **DEPRESSION**
Depression associated with severe phobias, such as claustrophobia or agoraphobia, may be treated with *Anacardium occ.* This state, in common with severe

exam nerves (*see above*), may manifest itself in a lack of self-confidence and a worsening of eczema in sufferers.

● **SKIN CONDITIONS**
Anacardium occ. is prescribed for skin conditions that itch, burn, or swell and become sore, or for blisters that may become infected. It may also be prescribed for leprosy, and to treat warts.

● **CAUTION**
The juice of *Anacardium occ.* is an irritant that causes blistering if it comes into contact with the skin. In 19th-century Europe it was used medicinally to burn off warts and corns.

APIS

Relieves the swelling of hives ◆ Helps ease
osteoarthritic pain ◆ Alleviates prostate problems

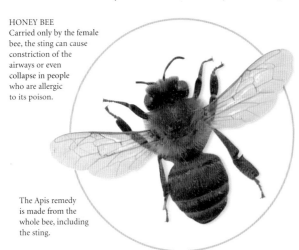

HONEY BEE
Carried only by the female
bee, the sting can cause
constriction of the
airways or even
collapse in people
who are allergic
to its poison.

One of the Apis
remedy's main
uses is to treat
insect stings.

The Apis remedy
is made from the
whole bee, including
the sting.

KEY ACTIONS

- PROVIDES RELIEF FROM ALLERGIES
- AIDS WITH FEELINGS OF JEALOUSY
- SOOTHES ANXIOUS RESTLESSNESS
- CURES CYSTITIS AND URINARY INFECTIONS

KEY PREPARATIONS

- TINCTURE made from the native European honey bee, which is now found in many parts of the world. The remedy is made from either the whole female bee, including the sting, or from the sting alone. The insect is crushed, dissolved in alcohol, diluted, and succussed.

INDICATIONS

● **PROSTATE PROBLEMS**
Prostitis (inflammation of the prostate) usually affects men in their thirties and forties; prostate cancer generally affects men over 60. *Apis* is indicated for an enlarged prostate with urine retention.

● **OSTEOARTHRITIS**
In some parts of the developed world, up to 90 percent of people over 40 have osteoarthritis. Severe osteoarthritis affects three times as many women as men. *Apis* is prescribed for inflammation of synovial membranes and overproduction of synovial fluids.

● **HIVES**
Also known as Urticaria, this condition consists of raised red patches – sometimes with paler centers – that itch intensely. It may be caused by food allergies, certain drugs, bites, stings, or stress. Treatment with *Apis* reduces the reaction.

● **ALLERGIES**
Apis is indicated as treatment for allergic swelling of the face, eyelids, lips, and mouth, and other inflammation.

● **URINARY INFECTIONS**
Cystitis, edema, and other urinary infections, including urine retention in newborn babies, can be treated with *Apis*.

37

ARGENTIUM NIT.

Prescribed for angina sufferers ◆ Eases Multiple Sclerosis

Relieves irritable bowel syndrome

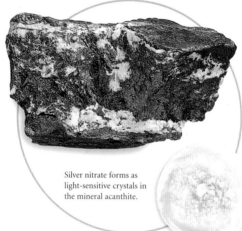

ACANTHITE

Acanthite is found in Norway, and North and South America.

The mineral acanthite is the main ore of silver.

Silver nitrate forms as light-sensitive crystals in the mineral acanthite.

SILVER NITRATE CRYSTALS

KEY ACTIONS

- CALMING
- CONTROLS THE INTESTINE
- USED TO TREAT WARTS
- AIDS THOSE WITH PHOBIAS

KEY PREPARATIONS

- TINCTURE made from pure crystals of silver nitrate dissolved in alcohol before being repeatedly diluted and succussed. *Argentum nit.* (silver nitrate) is found in acanthite, which usually occurs as crystals in hydrothermal veins in Norway, the U.S. and South America.

INDICATIONS

● **PHOBIAS**
Sufferers of multiple phobias associated with anxiety neuroses that originate in previous experiences may benefit from *Argentum nit.*

● **IRRITABLE BOWEL SYNDROME (IBS)**
Argentum nit. is indicated for irritation of the mucous membranes of the intestine and control of the gut by the autonomic nervous system.

● **MULTIPLE SCLEROSIS**
MS occurs if the myelin sheaths surrounding nerve fibers are damaged. *Argentum nit.* has a direct, qualitative effect upon nerves, controlling conscious movement.

● **ANGINA**
Argentum nit. is associated with improved nerve conduction to coronary arteries.

● **WARTS**
Argentum nit. was used for warts in the 19th century. It is still used in some wart medicines.

● **STRESS**
Argentum nit. is prescribed especially for exam stress.

● **CAUTION**
If ingested in large amounts, silver nitrate is highly poisonous.

ARNICA

Eases muscular pain, bruising, and sprains

Excellent first-aid remedy ◆ Helps control bleeding

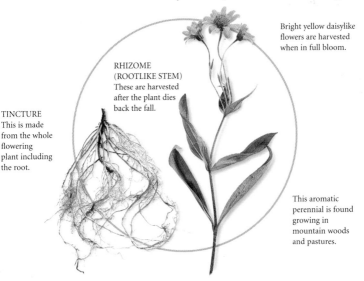

Bright yellow daisylike flowers are harvested when in full bloom.

RHIZOME (ROOTLIKE STEM) These are harvested after the plant dies back the fall.

TINCTURE This is made from the whole flowering plant including the root.

This aromatic perennial is found growing in mountain woods and pastures.

KEY ACTIONS

- PROMOTES TISSUE REPAIR
- ANTI-INFLAMMATORY
- TREATS GRIEF AND SHOCK
- EASES CRAMPS

KEY PREPARATIONS

- OINTMENT used externally to improve local blood supply and speed healing in the treatment of bruises, sprains, and muscle pain.
- TINCTURE made from the whole flowering plant, including the root. It is steeped in alcohol, filtered, diluted, and succussed.

INDICATIONS

● **SHOCK**
Dizziness after a fall or injury can be treated with *Arnica*. It also treats the early stages of grief, when the person displays signs of shock.

● **ERECTILE PROBLEMS**
Arnica is given to treat erectile dysfunction caused by bruising.

● **ANGINA**
Arnica is prescribed to heal damaged heart muscle, such as after a heart attack.

● **SKIN CONDITIONS**
Eczema and cracked, blistered nipples can be treated with *Arnica*.

● **FIRST AID**
Arnica is given following an accident, surgery, bereavement, childbirth, or dental treatment.

● **FEVER**
Recurring fevers, such as occur with typhoid or malarial fever, can be treated with *Arnica*.

● **CRAMPS**
Arnica relieves cramp. It is also prescribed for joint and muscular pain.

● **CAUTION**
Climbers used to chew, or drink an infusion of, *Arnica* leaves for aching muscles. Potentially toxic, its internal use is now mainly restricted to homeopathy.

BELLADONNA

Treats influenza and reduces fever

Eases menstrual pains ◆ Soothes painful, swollen breasts

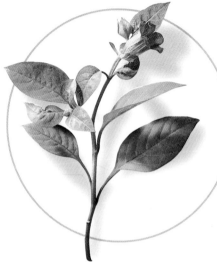

FLOWERS
Purple, bell-shaped flowers give way to black berries in the fall.

LEAVES
Leaves have a weaker effect than the root and for this reason are preferred for herbal medicines.

DEADLY NIGHTSHADE
Despite this plant's poisonous nature, it is used effectively in homeopathy.

KEY ACTIONS

- AIDS TEETHING INFANTS
- RELIEVES MASTITIS
- TREATS SUNSTROKE
- EASES KIDNEY PROBLEMS
- PRESCRIBED FOR ROSACEA

KEY PREPARATIONS

- TINCTURE made from the whole, fresh plant, including the root. As it comes into flower, the plant is dug up, chopped, and pounded to a pulp. The juice is then expressed and steeped in alcohol before being filtered, diluted, and succussed.

INDICATIONS

● **TEETHING**
Belladonna is prescribed to alleviate infant teething which is accompanied by sudden pain and a face that appears flushed.

● **ROSACEA**
Rosacea resembles mild adolescent acne. Its main feature is flushing of the skin. *Belladonna* is prescribed for the early stages, when the face is red, dry, and burning hot.

● **WOMEN'S PROBLEMS**
The remedy eases mastitis and menstrual pain.

● **FEVER**
Belladonna is a major remedy for acute illnesses

of sudden violent onset. It treats febrile convulsions and sunstroke.

● **ANESTHETIC**
Used in sleeping potions in Chaucer's time, today *Belladonna* provides an anesthetic still used in conventional medicine.

● **INFLUENZA**
Influenza with high fever (dilated pupils, flushed skin, throbbing pain) is treated with *Belladonna*.

● **KIDNEY PROBLEMS**
Belladonna treats cystitis and nephritis (inflamed kidneys).

● **CAUTION**
Belladonna is poisonous if taken in large amounts.

AURUM MET.

Prescribed for gland cancer ◆ Alleviates certain causes of infertility in men ◆ Treats circulatory problems

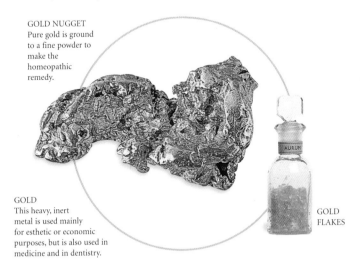

GOLD NUGGET
Pure gold is ground to a fine powder to make the homeopathic remedy.

GOLD
This heavy, inert metal is used mainly for esthetic or economic purposes, but is also used in medicine and in dentistry.

GOLD FLAKES

KEY ACTIONS

- HELPS WITH PHOBIAS
- TREATS REPRODUCTIVE DISORDERS
- CURES HEADACHES
- ALLEVIATES BONE PAINS
- PRESCRIBED FOR DEPRESSION AND GRIEF

KEY PREPARATIONS

- TINCTURE made from gold. The gold is purified from a nugget or extracted from an ore. It is then triturated with lactose sugar, filtered, diluted, and succussed.

INDICATIONS

● **CANCER**
There are many types of cancer and, as such, as wide a variety of remedies. *Aurum met.* is indicated for cancer of the glands.

● **MALE INFERTILITY**
There are several causes of male infertility, such as malformation of the testes or problems with the testicles (vas deferens). *Aurum met.* treats childhood atrophy of the testes and painful, swollen testicles.

● **PHOBIAS**
Homeopaths examine the physical symptoms that accompany phobias before prescribing a specific remedy; *Aurum met* is one indicated.

● **ARTHRITIS**
Aurum met. can help with the treatment of rheumatoid arthritis, a condition whereby the body's immune system attacks the joints. The remedy is indicated for destruction of the bone.

● **CIRCULATION**
Aurum met. is prescribed for circulatory problems, such as palpitations and angina.

● **CAUTION**
If any palpitations are severe, prolonged, or are accompanied by chest pains, consult a doctor.

BARYTA CARB.

Assists in stroke victims' recovery ◆ Lessens senile
dementia ◆ Treats prostate problems and impotence

BARIUM
CARBONATE
White crystals
are odorless
and toxic.

WHITE CRYSTALS
of barite and witherite
are found together.

The crystals are
ground into
powder to make
the homeopathic
remedy.

Barium is an element
found in the earth's
crust in minerals
such as barite and
witherite.

KEY ACTIONS

- TREATS IMPOTENCE
- INDICATED FOR ANXIETY
  AND PHOBIAS
- USED FOR RECURRENT
  COLDS
- HELPS WITH DOWN'S
  SYNDROME
- PRESCRIBED TO EASE
  CONFUSION

KEY PREPARATIONS

- POWDER made from
  crystals of barium
  carbonate that have
  been chemically
  prepared (barium
  chloride precipitated
  with a weak solution
  of ammonia). The
  crystals are mixed
  with lactose sugar
  and triturated.

INDICATIONS

● **PROSTATE PROBLEMS**
Baryta carb. is prescribed
when the patient has a
frequent urge to urinate,
produces only a slow
stream of urine, or when
impotence occurs.

● **DEVELOPMENTAL
PROBLEMS**
The remedy is given for
senile dementia in the
elderly and mental
confusion. It is also given
to improve slow physical
or mental development in
children, and for people
with Down's syndrome.

● **STROKE**
Stroke occurs when the
blood supply to part of
the brain is interrupted or

insufficient. Strokes are
more likely to affect men
than women, and
incidence increases
sharply with age. As
symptoms and sufferers
vary, there are several
homeopathic remedies for
stroke. *Baryta carb.* is
suitable to treat the very
elderly and the physically
and mentally weak.

● **COUGHS & COLDS**
Baryta carb. is indicated
for recurrent colds and
coughs, sore throats, and
swollen tonsils.

● **CAUTION**
Barium carbonate is
a powerful poison.
Non-homeopathic
doses cause nausea
and vomiting.

BRYONIA

Eases painful breasts ◆ Alleviates constipation

Treats coughs and bronchitis

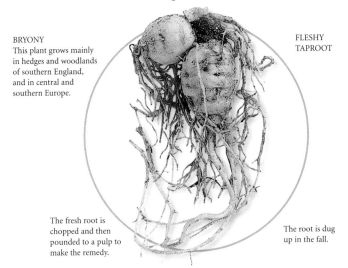

BRYONY
This plant grows mainly in hedges and woodlands of southern England, and in central and southern Europe.

FLESHY TAPROOT

The fresh root is chopped and then pounded to a pulp to make the remedy.

The root is dug up in the fall.

KEY ACTIONS

- RELIEVES SORE BREASTS
- EASES CHEST PROBLEMS
- RELIEVES PAIN
- EASES INFLAMMATION

KEY PREPARATIONS

- TINCTURE made from the fresh root. It is unearthed before the plant flowers, chopped, pulped, macerated in alcohol for 10 days, diluted, and succussed.

INDICATIONS

● **PAIN RELIEF**
The chief physical symptom treated by *Bryonia* is pain felt on the slightest movement. This includes bad headaches and rheumatic pain.

● **CONSTIPATION**
Bryonia is indicated for constipation where the sufferer eventually passes dry, hard stools and has dry mucous membranes.

● **CHEST PROBLEMS**
Bryonia eases a variety of chest problems, including coughing accompanied by chest pain or fever. It is also prescribed to reduce internal inflammation of the chest, for pneumonia, for shortness of breath, and to clear phlegm.

● **BRONCHITIS**
Bryonia treats patients suffering from bronchitis which is accompanied by a painful cough.

● **BREAST PROBLEMS**
For hard, inflamed breasts, which are painful on every movement (such as before a period), bryonia may be taken regularly for up to a maximum of five days.

● **CAUTION**
Used externally, the fresh root of *Bryonia* can cause severe skin irritation. Non-homeopathic doses can cause death within hours.

CALC. CARB.

Treats chronic fatigue syndrome (CFS)

Inhibits uterine fibroids ◆ Eases asthma

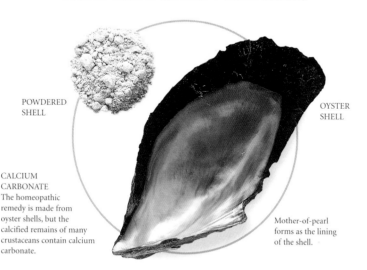

POWDERED
SHELL

OYSTER
SHELL

CALCIUM
CARBONATE
The homeopathic
remedy is made from
oyster shells, but the
calcified remains of many
crustaceans contain calcium
carbonate.

Mother-of-pearl
forms as the lining
of the shell.

KEY ACTIONS

- TREATS ECZEMA
- CALMS PALPITATIONS
- EASES ANXIETY
- PROMOTES GOOD
  DIGESTION
- HELPS WITH DENTAL
  PROBLEMS
- RELIEVES HEADACHES

KEY PREPARATIONS

- POWDERED SHELL
  made from
  mother-of-pearl,
  secreted by oysters.
  The mother-of-pearl
  is removed from the
  outer shell. It is
  cleaned, dried, and
  triturated with
  lactose sugar.

INDICATIONS

● **ANXIETY**
Calc. carb. is prescribed
for anxiety-related
conditions and phobias,
particularly those that
may escalate into
obsessive behavior.

● **ECZEMA**
The cause of eczema is
often unknown and
symptoms vary. The
homeopath will want to
know a full medical
history, including that of
the patient's family, and
any possible triggers. *Calc.
carb.* is one remedy given.

● **CHEST PROBLEMS**
Asthma, and other
ailments arising out of
restricted movement of

the ribcage, are treated
with *Calc. carb.*

● **PALPITATIONS**
Not all palpitations are
serious, but they should
always be investigated by
a doctor. *Calc. carb.* is
among several remedies
recommended by
homeopaths.

● **CHRONIC FATIGUE
SYNDROME (CFS)**
Calc. carb. treats fatigue,
particularly of the thigh
muscles, from walking.

● **FIBROIDS**
Fibroids are benign (non-
cancerous) growths. *Calc.
carb.* is used for the
treatment of these
growths that project from
the uterine wall.

CALC. PHOS.

Relieves painful breasts ◆ Maintains strong bones

Eases the symptoms of rheumatoid arthritis

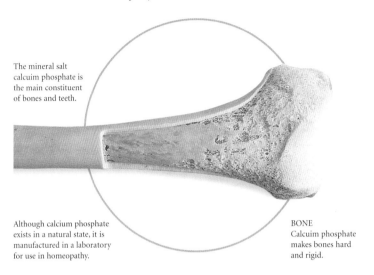

The mineral salt calcium phosphate is the main constituent of bones and teeth.

Although calcium phosphate exists in a natural state, it is manufactured in a laboratory for use in homeopathy.

BONE
Calcuim phosphate makes bones hard and rigid.

KEY ACTIONS

- TREATS ROSACEA
- PRESCRIBED TO HELP PHOBIAS
- EASES TEETHING PROBLEMS
- PROMOTES GOOD DIGESTION

KEY PREPARATIONS

- MINERAL SALTS made from white calcium phosphate precipitate. It is filtered, dried, and triturated with lactose sugar.

INDICATIONS

● **BONES**
Calcium and phosphorus are essential to bone maintenance. *Calc. phos.* treats conditions such as slow-healing fractures, joint disorders, and slow growth in children.

● **DIGESTIVE DISORDERS**
Calc. phos. promotes good digestion in those who find it difficult to eat, due perhaps to cramps, pain, nausea, or diarrhea.

● **ARTHRITIS**
This remedy is used to treat rheumatoid arthritis. *Calc. phos.* affects the maintenance of bones and is given if they are soft, thin, and brittle.

● **ROSACEA**
Calc. phos. is prescribed for rosacea that is found mainly on the nose, and is accompanied by pimples.

● **PHOBIAS**
There are many types of phobia; *Calc. phos.* is often used to treat those centered around school.

● **BREAST PROBLEMS**
Calc. phos. is given for painful breast lumps and swelling.

● **TEETH**
Teething problems and weak teeth are treated with *Calc. phos.*

● **FATIGUE**
Calc. phos. is indicated for fatigue and anemia.

CANTHARIS

Key treatment for intestinal disorders

Treats kidney problems ◆ Eases cystitis

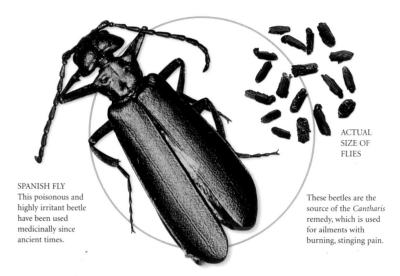

SPANISH FLY
This poisonous and highly irritant beetle have been used medicinally since ancient times.

ACTUAL SIZE OF FLIES

These beetles are the source of the *Cantharis* remedy, which is used for ailments with burning, stinging pain.

KEY ACTIONS

- RELIEVES PAIN
- EASES INFLAMMATION
- CONTROLS EXCESSIVE LIBIDO
- TREATS URINARY DISORDERS
- PROMOTES GOOD DIGESTION

KEY PREPARATIONS

- TINCTURE made from whole, live beetles. They are heated, macerated in alcohol, and left to stand for 5 days. They are then filtered, diluted, and succussed.

INDICATIONS

● KIDNEYS

Cantharis is given for tenderness in the kidneys, for renal colic, and kidney inflammation.

● ULCERATIVE COLITIS

Ulcerative colitis is an inflammatory bowel disease in which the linings of the rectum and colon gradually become more ulcerated. *Cantharis* reduces inflammation of the gut lining and the production of mucus.

● EXCESSIVE LIBIDO

Often claimed as aphrodisiac, *Cantharis* is given for uncontrollable, inappropriate sexual arousal.

● CYSTITIS

Cystitis affects mainly women, but can be present in men. Regular doses of *Cantharis* are prescribed.

● IRRITABLE BOWEL SYNDROME (IBS)

Inflammation of the gastrointestinal tract, especially the lower bowel, is treated with *Cantharis*.

● CAUTION

This beetle secretes cantharidine if touched. This chemical causes the skin to blister. Non-homeopathic doses can cause severe damage to the urinary system.

CARBO VEG.

Alleviates symptoms of chronic fatigue syndrome (C...

Eases indigestion ◆ Reduces bloating

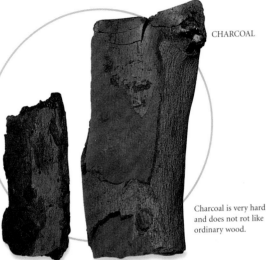

Woods from different trees make charcoal with different properties. Silver birch, beech, or poplar trees are used in homepathy.

CHARCOAL

CHARCOAL
Wood is burned in a sealed environment from which air is excluded to make charcoal.

Charcoal is very hard and does not rot like ordinary wood.

KEY ACTIONS

- RELIEVES FLATULENCE
- TREATS FATIGUE
- DISINFECTS
- IMPROVES CIRCULATION
- AIDS BREATHING

KEY PREPARATIONS

- TINCTURE made from the wood of the silver birch, beech, or poplar trees. Fist-sized pieces of wood are cut, heated until red hot, and sealed in an airtight earthenware jar. The resulting ash is then triturated, diluted, and succussed.

INDICATIONS

● **CHRONIC FATIGUE SYNDROME (CFS)**
Carbo veg. alleviates the aches and burning pains throughout the body that are associated with CFS.

● **BLOATING**
Bloating and flatulence may be due to constipation or intestinal problems. If the condition is relieved by burping, a homeopath may recommend *Carbo veg.*

● **INDIGESTION**
For indigestion with excessive flatulence, especially that which occurs regardless of the patient's diet, *Carbo veg.* should be taken regularly.

It is also prescribed for those with a sluggish digestive system, particularly elderly patients.

● **ANTISEPTIC**
Used throughout history as a "purifier." In the 18th and 19th centuries *Carbo veg.* was used in dressings for wounds and in some mouthwashes. It is used in both traditional and conventional medicine for ulceration and septic diseases, and is known for its deodorant and disinfectant properties.

● **BREATHING TROUBLE**
Used to treat spasmodic coughs, whooping cough, asthma, and bronchitis in the elderly.

CAUSTICUM

Improves nerve and muscle function

Cures bedwetting • Treats warts

This compound is not used in any form of medicine other than homeopathy.

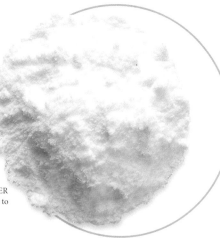

POTASIUM HYDRATE
Slaked lime and sulfate of potash are dissolved in purified water to make the causticum tincture.

POTASIUM HYDRATE POWDER
The powder is used to make a solution of slaked lime.

KEY ACTIONS

- RELIEVES BURNS
- TREATS BELL'S PALSY AND MULTIPLE SCLEROSIS
- PROMOTES SKIN HEALING
- CURES LARYNGITIS

KEY PREPARATIONS

- TINCTURE made from slaked lime and sulfate of potash. They are combined and dissolved in purified water. This solution is then further diluted and succussed.

INDICATIONS

● **MULTIPLE SCLEROSIS**
Causticum is indicated for progressive debilitation of the nervous system.

● **MUSCLE WEAKNESS**
Causticum is most often prescribed for weakness, which may progress to paralysis, of the nerves and muscles, especially of the bladder, larynx, vocal cords, upper eyelids, and the right side of the face. Muscle weakness may show both as twitching and as stiffness that causes mobility problems.

● **WARTS**
For warts that occur near the nails, or on the feet or face or eyelids, a course of

Causticum, lasting approximately three weeks, may be given.

● **FIRST AID**
Causticum is a first aid remedy for severe burns.

● **SKIN CONDITIONS**
Slow-healing burns, scars, and blisters, as well as boils, eczema, herpes, and acne may benefit from using *Causticum*.

● **LARYNGITIS**
Use *Causticum* for laryngitis with a dry, raw throat and violent cough.

● **BEDWETTING**
Causticum, taken before bed, cures bedwetting that occurs soon after the patient falls asleep.

IPECAC.

Relieves morning sickness ◆ Stems heavy
menstrual bleeding ◆ Alleviates general nausea

The plant grows in
South America,
mainly in Brazil.

IPECACUANHA
A traditional
Brazilian cure for
dysentery that was
taken to Europe in
1672 and is
still used today
by herbalists for
amebic dysentery.

The root of 3-year-
old plants are
unearthed when the
plant is in flower
and dried to make
the remedy.

DRIED
ROOT

KEY ACTIONS

- EASES WHEEZING AND
  ASTHMA
- TREATS NOSEBLEEDS
- RELIEVES COUGHS
- TREATS HEAVY
  BLEEDING

KEY PREPARATIONS

- TINCTURE made from
  the root. It is dug up,
  and the firmest,
  darkest rootlets are
  dried, powdered,
  and macerated in
  alcohol. They are
  then filtered, diluted,
  and succussed.

INDICATIONS

● **NAUSEA**
Persistent nausea, with or
without vomiting, is
treated with *Ipecac.* For
constant nausea, possibly
accompanied by
headaches, perspiration,
and diarrhea, *Ipecac.*
should be taken regularly.

● **ASTHMA**
The remedy is prescribed
for patients whose asthma
attacks are accompanied
by persistent nausea.

● **COUGHS & WHEEZING**
Ipecac. is prescribed for
coughing fits that cause
wheezing, breathing
difficulties, and a
constricted chest. It is
effective in treating

irritating, dry, rattling
loose coughs, and those
triggered by warm or
humid weather.

● **MORNING SICKNESS**
Ipecac. may be prescribed
for morning sickness
where, despite vomiting,
the tongue remains clean
and unfurred.

● **BLEEDING**
Ipecac. is prescribed to
treat nosebleeds and
heavy menstrual bleeding.
It is also given to patients
with a tendency to bleed
easily.

● **CAUTION**
Non-homeopathic doses,
of *Ipecac.* cause nausea
and vomiting; they may
lead to cardiac failure.

49

CHAMOMILLA

Cures sleeplessness ● Calms irritability in children
and adults ● Treats toothache and earache

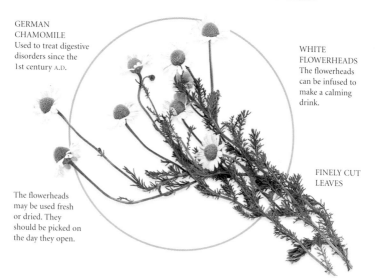

GERMAN
CHAMOMILE
Used to treat digestive
disorders since the
1st century A.D.

WHITE
FLOWERHEADS
The flowerheads
can be infused to
make a calming
drink.

FINELY CUT
LEAVES

The flowerheads
may be used fresh
or dried. They
should be picked on
the day they open.

KEY ACTIONS

- CALMS
- SOOTHES
- RELIEVES PAIN
- ASSISTS WITH LABOR
  AND MENSTRUAL PAINS

KEY PREPARATIONS

- TINCTURE made from
  the whole, fresh
  plant, harvested
  when in flower. It is
  finely chopped and
  macerated in alcohol
  before being diluted
  and succussed.

INDICATIONS

● **CHILDREN'S HEALTH**
Chamomilla is often given
to children who are
snappy, wail when ill, and
are pacified only by being
held. It is prescribed for
teething with irritability
and anger, and for temper
tantrums when the child
is impossible to please.

● **TOOTHACHE**
Toothache accompanied
by unbearable pain, such
as when an abscess occurs,
can be treated with
Chamomilla.

● **PAIN RELIEF**
Chamomilla provides
relief from pain which
seems unbearable.
Symptoms it can alleviate

include excruciating
earache accompanied by
fever; stomach pain with
diarrhea; colic; and
swollen glands causing
facial and neck pain.

● **WOMEN'S HEALTH**
Women's health problems
alleviated by *Chamomilla*
include menstrual pains
which induce sweats,
anger, or fainting; labor
pains; inflamed nipples;
and pain from breast-
feeding, causing anger in
the mother.

● **SLEEPLESSNESS**
A course of *Chamomilla*
reduces sleeplessness
caused by anger and
irritability. Drinking
chamomile tea before bed
also promotes good sleep.

50

CHELIDONIUM

Treats liver problems ◈ Prepares the body
for surgery ◈ Eases lung complaints

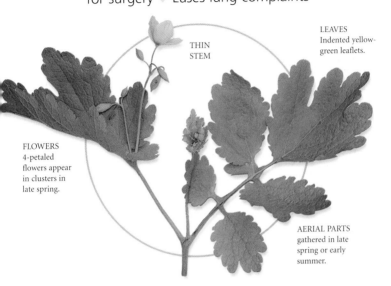

THIN
STEM

LEAVES
Indented yellow-
green leaflets.

FLOWERS
4-petaled
flowers appear
in clusters in
late spring.

AERIAL PARTS
gathered in late
spring or early
summer.

KEY ACTIONS

- RELAXES MUSCLES
- RELIEVES PAIN
- TREATS GALLSTONES
- TREATS PNEUMONIA

KEY PREPARATIONS

- TINCTURE made from either the whole flowering plant, or just the root. It is chopped, pulped, and macerated in alcohol for at least 10 days.

INDICATIONS

● **PREOPERATIVE CARE**
Chelidonium may be given prior to surgery for hepatitis or gallstones.

● **LIVER PROBLEMS**
Chelidonium is associated with liver problems, as well as those arising from the spleen, kidney, and intestine. It is effective in treating hepatitis.

● **GALLBLADDER**
This remedy is used in traditional medicine for problems arising from the gallbladder. Patients with gallstones feel pain on the upper right side of the abdomen – *Chelidonium* is associated with right-sided symptoms.

● **PAIN RELIEF**
Chelidonium is a muscle relaxant and, as such, useful for relieving pain, such as headaches that occur on the right side of the head, backache, and shoulder pain.

● **LUNGS**
Pneumonia, especially that which chiefly affects the right lung, and other lung complaints may be treated with *Chelidonium*.

● **EYES**
Dioscorides, the famous Greek physician from the 1st century A.D., prescribed *Chelidonium* for eye problems and to sharpen the eyesight. Western and Chinese herbalists use it to treat cataracts.

CHINA

Treats malaria ◆ Relieves chronic fatigue syndrome (CFS) ◆ Treats exhaustion

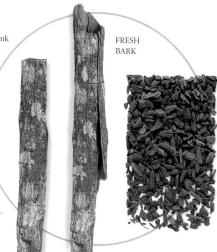

The bark of the trunk is most commonly used medicinally.

FRESH BARK

PERUVIAN BARK
In the 17th century, Jesuits used quinine extracted from Peruvian bark, as a cure for malaria. It was widely adopted in Europe as a treatment for fevers.

DRIED BARK

KEY ACTIONS

- RELIEVES INSOMNIA
- HELPS REPLENISH LOST FLUIDS
- TREATS FEVER
- EASES HEADACHES
- PRELIEVES INDIGESTION

KEY PREPARATIONS

- TINCTURE made from dried Peruvian bark. It is macerated in alcohol for at least five days before being filtered, diluted, and then succussed.

INDICATIONS

● MALARIA
This bark is of particular historical significance for homeopaths, since quinine extracted from it became the subject of Hahnemann's first homeopathic proving. Today the remedy is a key treatment for malarial symptoms.

● HEADACHES
China treats throbbing pains in the head, possibly linked to facial neuralgia, nosebleeds, tinnitus, or liver disorders.

● CHRONIC FATIGUE SYNDROME (CFS)
China is prescribed to CFS sufferers to help combat bloating, anxiety, sleeplessness, and a feeling of weakness after the slightest exertion.

● EXHAUSTION
The remedy is used for exhaustion following illness or extreme fluid loss.

● INSOMNIA
Sleeplessness due to excited thoughts, where even the slightest noise disrupts the sleeper, can be treated with *China*.

● CAUTION
If taken in non-homeopathic doses, quinine causes harmful symptoms similar to those of malaria.

COFFEA

Relieves pain ◆ Treats insomnia
Cures headaches and toothache

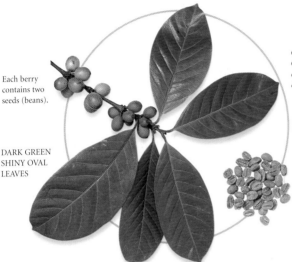

COFFEE
Coffee's stimulating effect is weakened if drunk repeatedly.

Each berry contains two seeds (beans).

DARK GREEN SHINY OVAL LEAVES

COFFEE BEANS
The best quality beans are produced by fermenting, sun-drying, and roasting seeds.

KEY ACTIONS

- CURES PALPITATIONS
- REDUCES OVER-EXCITEMENT
- RELIEVES MENOPAUSAL FLUSHES
- RELIEVES PAIN

KEY PREPARATIONS

- TINCTURE made from ripe, unroasted coffee beans. These are macerated in alcohol for at least five days before being filtered. The resulting liquid is then repeatedly diluted and succussed.

INDICATIONS

● **PAIN RELIEF**
In modern medicine, caffeine is combined with conventional analgesics, such as aspirin, to make over-the-counter painkillers. *Coffea* is recommended for hypersensitivity to pain, to the point where pain causes intense despair.

● **INSOMNIA**
Coffea can help combat insomnia, particularly that which derives from an inability to relax.

● **HEADACHES**
Coffea is prescribed for one-sided pain in the head which feels as if a nail is being driven into it, and for pain that sets in upon waking and can seem unbearable. Ayurvedic medicine uses unripe beans to treat headaches.

● **TOOTHACHE**
For toothache with severe, shooting pain – that often shoots from the teeth to the tips of the fingers – take *Coffea* daily.

● **OVEREXCITEMENT**
Coffea is prescribed to reduce overexcitement and calm palpitations.

● **CAUTION**
Non-homeopathic doses of caffeine upset digestion, drains the body of calcium, and can cause nervousness.

CONIUM

Eases mental strain ◆ Treats prostate problems
Relieves breast pain

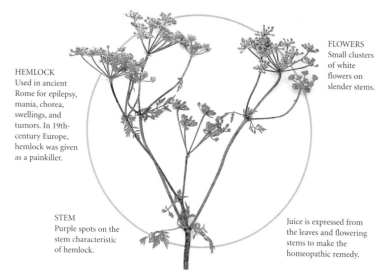

HEMLOCK
Used in ancient Rome for epilepsy, mania, chorea, swellings, and tumors. In 19th-century Europe, hemlock was given as a painkiller.

FLOWERS
Small clusters of white flowers on slender stems.

STEM
Purple spots on the stem characteristic of hemlock.

Juice is expressed from the leaves and flowering stems to make the homeopathic remedy.

KEY ACTIONS

- COUNTERS PREMATURE AGING
- TREATS CYSTS
- RELIEVES MENTAL STRAIN
- RESTORES VITALITY

KEY PREPARATIONS

- TINCTURE made from the fresh flowering plant, including the root. It is macerated in alcohol, diluted, and succussed.

INDICATIONS

● TUMORS
Breast lumps mainly occur in women aged between 30 and 50; 80 per cent are benign, but all should be investigated by a doctor. Hard breast tumors are treated with *Conium* – it was used for breast tumors in the 1st century A.D. It is also indicated for treatment of tumors or cysts in the reproductive organs.

● MENTAL STRAIN
Conium treats illnesses caused by mental strain or grief.

● PROSTATE PROBLEMS
Conium is given for an enlarged prostate, particularly when a discharge of prostatic fluid occurs.

● BREAST PAIN
Conium is prescribed for breast pain, especially that which occurs when the breast is tender even when touched lightly.

● THE ELDERLY
In the elderly, *Conium* is thought to restore vitality; it is also believed to counter premature aging.

● CAUTION
Non-homeopathic doses of this plant can cause paralysis, primarily of the respiratory nerves. This can therefore lead to death caused by suffocation.

COLOCYNTHIS

Treats irritable bowel syndrome

Treats gastroenteritis ◆ Relieves sciatica

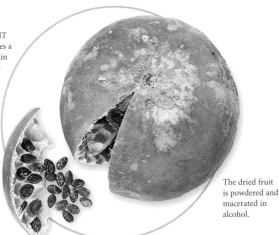

DRIED FRUIT
This resembles a
small pumpkin
the size of an
orange.

SEEDS
These are
considered
nutritious, but
are not used in
homeopathy.

The dried fruit
is powdered and
macerated in
alcohol.

KEY ACTIONS

- RELIEVES PAIN
- TREATS ULCERATIVE COLITIS
- RELIEVES SCIATICA
- CURES COLIC

KEY PREPARATIONS

- TINCTURE made from the dried, deseeded fruit. It is powdered and macerated in alcohol before being diluted and succussed.

INDICATIONS

● **PAIN RELIEF**
Colocynthis is given for the relief of acute pain and especially for: colicky abdominal pain; cramping in the hips, kidneys, and ovaries; headaches; or shooting nerve pain in the face, neck, and limbs. It may also be prescribed for gout and for rheumatic pain in the neck.

● **GASTROENTERITIS**
Gastroenteritis where the patient suffers severe abdominal cramps can be treated with *Colocynthis*.

● **SCIATICA**
There are several homeopathic remedies for different forms of sciatica. *Colocynthis* treats that which worsens in cold, damp weather.

● **IRRITABLE BOWEL SYNDROME (IBS)**
The remedy treats griping pains that are relieved when the patient bends double or applies pressure to the abdomen.

● **COLIC**
Colocynthis is indicated for colic with severe pains.

● **CAUTION**
This is a bitter gourd that contains a substance called colocynthin. Non-homeopathic doses cause severe cramps and gastrointestinal inflammation.

CUPRUM MET.

Cures cramps in the extremities and stomach

Eases physical and mental exhaustion ◆ Treats convulsions

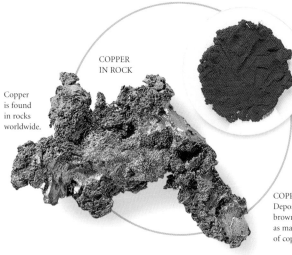

COPPER
IN ROCK

Copper
is found
in rocks
worldwide.

POWDERED
COPPER
Copper is
powdered to
make the
homeopathic
remedy.

COPPER
Deposits of this reddish-
brown mineral are found
as massive or thin sheets
of copper.

KEY ACTIONS

- RELAXES MUSCLES
- RELIEVES PAIN
- ALLEVIATES COLICKY
  CONDITIONS

KEY PREPARATIONS

- TINCTURE made from
  powdered copper.
  The metal is
  triturated with
  lactose sugar, then
  ground repeatedly
  until it forms a
  water-soluble
  powder. It is filtered,
  diluted, and
  succussed.

INDICATIONS

● **CRAMPS**
This occurs when the
muscles go into spasm as
a result of shortage of
oxygen or from a build-
up of lactic acid. *Cuprum
met.* is indicated primarily
for severe cramps in the
legs, fingers, or feet.

● **CONVULSIONS**
Cuprum met. is given for
convulsions, including
those linked to epilepsy
and those experienced by
very young children.

● **EXHAUSTION**
The remedy is prescribed
to relieve exhaustion,
perhaps following illness,
lack of sleep, or severe
mental strain. Symptoms

may include cramps and
headaches between the
eyes. The remedy is linked
to the nervous system.

● **DIGESTION**
Cuprum met. is chiefly
associated with the
digestive system,
especially with alleviating
stomach cramps. It is
effective in easing
spasmodic, colicky pains,
when the abdomen is hot,
tender, and sore.

● **CAUTION**
Although used by
doctors as late as the
1880s in ointments for
healing wounds, non-
homeopathic doses of
copper are toxic and can
cause convulsions,
paralysis, and even death.

56

STAPHYSAGRIA

Treats urogenital problems ◆ Cures insomnia

Relieves headaches and toothache

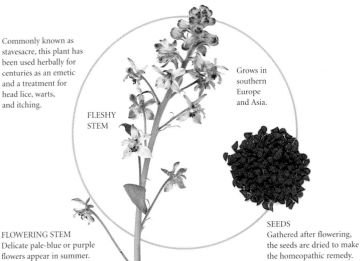

Commonly known as stavesacre, this plant has been used herbally for centuries as an emetic and a treatment for head lice, warts, and itching.

Grows in southern Europe and Asia.

FLESHY STEM

FLOWERING STEM
Delicate pale-blue or purple flowers appear in summer.

SEEDS
Gathered after flowering, the seeds are dried to make the homeopathic remedy.

KEY ACTIONS

- CALMS PALPITATIONS
- TREATS PAINFUL SKIN CONDITIONS
- SOOTHES SORE EYES
- EASES GRIEF
- TREATS INFERTILITY IN IWOMEN

KEY PREPARATIONS

- TINCTURE The seeds of the plant are gathered once it has finished flowering. They are dried, triturated, and succussed.

INDICATIONS

● **INFERTILITY**
Provided there are no physiological problems, constitutional treatment will try to rectify imbalances in the body systems controlling reproduction. Remedies are determined largely by an individual's symptoms. *Staphisagria* is associated with women.

● **GRIEF**
Staphisagria is indicated for suppressed grief, linked to embarrassment or humiliation.

● **SKIN CONDITIONS**
Staphisagria is used to treat skin conditions that are affected by irritability

of the nervous system, such as psoriasis.

● **VAGINISMUS**
An unusual condition in which the muscles surrounding the entrance of the vagina go into spasm, making sexual intercourse, medical examination, or the use of tampons painful or impossible. *Staphisagria* is prescribed for vaginismus that occurs after medical examination.

● **EYES**
The remedy soothes inflamed, painful eyes and treats styes.

● **CAUTION**
Non-homeopathic doses can be poisonous.

57

DIOSCOREA

Treats menstrual problems ◆ Treats renal colic
and kidney stones ◆ Key remedy for severe pains

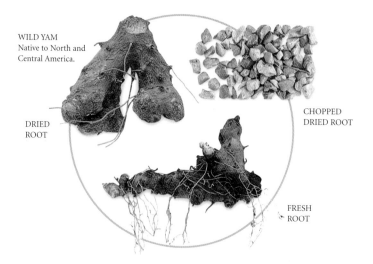

WILD YAM
Native to North and
Central America.

CHOPPED
DRIED ROOT

DRIED
ROOT

FRESH
ROOT

KEY ACTIONS

- RELIEVES PAIN
- TREATS NEURALGIA
- TREATS COLIC
- ALLEVIATES LIVER
  PROBLEMS

KEY PREPARATIONS

- TINCTURE made from
  the fresh root, dug
  up after the plant
  has flowered. It is
  chopped and
  macerated in alcohol.

INDICATIONS

● COLIC
Dioscorea (wild yam), a
traditional Aztec remedy
for pain, was used in
Central America for colic.
Today it is prescribed for
colicky pains, and for
neuralgic pains of the
gastrointestinal system.

● WOMEN'S HEALTH
Used by the Aztecs for
menstrual pain, and still
given for menstruation
problems. *Dioscorea* was
also used in production of
the first contraceptive pill.

● MEN'S HEALTH
In men, *Dioscorea* is
typically prescribed to
treat renal colic associated
with kidney stones, sharp

pains radiating down the
testicles and legs, and
where cold, clammy
perspiration is present.

● PAIN RELIEF
Dioscorea is indicated for
pains that are severe,
cutting, cramping, and
grinding, and for those
that radiate out in all
directions from a central
point, which may shift in
location. The pains may
affect the area of the liver,
and radiate toward the
right nipple.

● CAUTION
Non-homeopathic doses
of wild yam should not
be taken without medical
advice by women who
are also taking the
contraceptive pill.

EUPHRASIA

Soothes conjunctivitis ◆ Eases general eye problems

Treats hay fever and other allergies

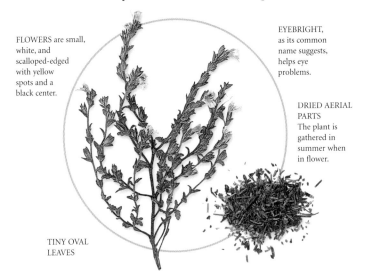

FLOWERS are small, white, and scalloped-edged with yellow spots and a black center.

EYEBRIGHT, as its common name suggests, helps eye problems.

DRIED AERIAL PARTS The plant is gathered in summer when in flower.

TINY OVAL LEAVES

KEY ACTIONS

- EASES INFLAMMATION
- SOOTHES IRRITATION
- REDUCES EYE STRAIN
- TREATS ALLERGIES

KEY PREPARATIONS

- TINCTURE made from the whole, fresh flowering plant, including the root. It is chopped and macerated in alcohol.

INDICATIONS

● **ALLERGIES**
The remedy is used mainly for allergies and infection affecting the eyes and nose, such as colds and hay fever, where the eyes are mainly affected. It is also indicated for allergies affecting the middle ear and sinuses.

● **EYE PROBLEMS**
Also known as eyebright, *Euphrasia* has a classic affinity to the eyes. It has been used to treat eye strain and inflammation since the Middle Ages. Today it is given for irritation with cutting, burning, pressing pains and sticky mucus; when

eyes have a heightened sensitivity to light, with burning, swollen eyelids and frequent blinking; and when eyes water profusely. It may also be prescribed for eye symptoms that occur after an injury.

● **CONJUNCTIVITIS**
Inflammation of the conjunctiva results either from infection (yellow discharge) or allergy (whites of the eyes are red and gritty). Conjunctivitis is typified by the presence of swollen eyelids with a burning discharge and a frequent need to blink. In some cases, little blisters may form inside the eyelids. *Euphrasia* is the usual remedy prescribed.

SPONGIA

Treats heart problems ◆ Eases respiratory trouble

Eases certain phobias

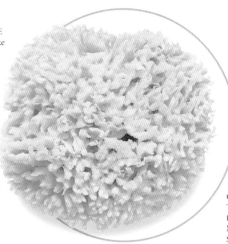

FRESH SPONGE is roasted to make a remedy for swelling of the thyroid glands and coughs.

COMMON SPONGE Traditionally gathered from the waters of the Mediterranean, near Syria and Greece.

KEY ACTIONS

- EASES INFLAMMATION
- CALMING
- TREATS THYROID PROBLEMS
- FIGHTS INFECTION
- REDUCES PALPITATIONS

KEY PREPARATIONS

- TINCTURE The sponge is carefully cleaned of sand, then toasted in a metal drum before being powdered and triturated.

INDICATIONS

● **PHOBIAS**
Spongia (the common sponge) is appropriate for those who have a marked fear of heart disease and of death, particularly by suffocation. They may feel uncomfortable in clothes.

● **HEART PROBLEMS**
There is a strong focus on the heart with *Spongia*. Typical symptoms include palpitations or an uneasy feeling in the area of the heart. Congestion may result, with a sensation as though blood is rushing into the chest and face. A fear of suffocation and a sense of the heart being forced upward can disrupt sleep. Other

symptoms include exhaustion and the body feeling heavy, so that even slight exertion causes prostration.

● **RESPIRATION**
Spongia is prescribed for upper-respiratory-tract infections that tend to settle in the larynx, such as a dry, hollow, croupy cough. There is typically a feeling of dryness in the mucous membranes, and pain in the larynx that worsens with swallowing, singing, or talking.

● **GLANDS**
Inflammation, hardening, and enlargement of the glands, especially the thyroid, can be treated effectively with *Spongia*.

FERRUM PHOS.

Treats urogenital problems ◆ Relieves digestive disorders

Assists sufferers of Raynaud's disease

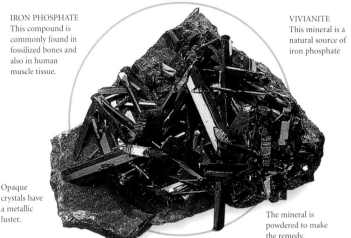

IRON PHOSPHATE
This compound is commonly found in fossilized bones and also in human muscle tissue.

VIVIANITE
This mineral is a natural source of iron phosphate

Opaque crystals have a metallic luster.

The mineral is powdered to make the remedy.

KEY ACTIONS

- FIGHTS INFECTION
- IMPROVES CIRCULATION
- HELPS RESTORE MALE LIBIDO
- EASES INFLAMMATION
- REDUCES FEVER

KEY PREPARATIONS

- TINCTURE prepared chemically from iron sulfate, sodium phosphate, and sodium acetate. The powdered mineral is triturated. Although it is chemically prepared for homeopathy, iron phosphate occurs naturally in vivianite.

INDICATIONS

● **COLDS**
Colds are caused by viral infections of the respiratory tract. A neglected cold may infect the chest, ears, throat, sinuses, or larynx. As such, it is important to treat the early signs of a cold. *Ferrum phos.* may be prescribed for a cold that comes on slowly.

● **FEVER**
Ferrum phos. fights infection at the early stages and reduces fever.

● **DIGESTIVE PROBLEMS**
Indigestion, sour burps, and vomiting of food that appears not to have been properly digested may be

treated with *Ferrum phos.* It may also be given for irritable bowel syndrome or constipation.

● **MEN'S HEALTH**
Used to treat a marked loss of libido in men.

● **WOMEN'S HEALTH**
Ferrum phos. is used to treat uterine pain, a short menstrual cycle, vaginal dryness, and nocturnal stress incontinence in women.

● **RAYNAUD'S DISEASE**
This is due to restricted blood flow when the blood vessels contract in the cold. *Ferrum phos.* is prescribed for this and other problems associated with poor circulation.

GELSEMIUM

Treats neurological disorders ◆ Reduces fever

Calms phobias and anticipatory fears

CAROLINA JASMINE
This came into regular
use from the middle of
the 19th century, chiefly
as a treatment for
nervous disorders
such as sciatica and
neuralgia.

Fresh root
gives off an
aromatic odor.

ROOTSTOCK
This is unearthed
in the fall, and the
fresh root is used
to make
homeopathic
remedies.

The fresh root
is bitter and
extremely toxic.

KEY ACTIONS

- CALMS STAGE FRIGHT
  AND EXAM NERVES
- TREATS SCIATICA
- EASES INFLUENZA
- HELPS HAY FEVER
  SUFFERERS

KEY PREPARATIONS

- TINCTURE made from
  the fresh bark of the
  root. It is finely
  chopped and
  macerated in alcohol.

INDICATIONS

● **FEARS**
Gelsemium is often used
to combat phobias, exam
nerves, stage fright, and
other anticipatory terrors.
At times the remedy has
been given to strengthen
courage on the battlefield.

● **NEUROLOGY**
A general state of physical
and/or mental paralysis,
with weakness and an
inability to perform, are
key symptoms linked to
this remedy. Certain
anticipatory terrors (*see
above*) cause trembling,
weakness, diarrhea, and
frequent urination; in the
long term, these may lead
to more complicated
serious neurological

disorders, possibly even
paralysis, which the
remedy may help. It has
been used to treat
neuralgia, sciatica, and
other nervous disorders
since the middle of the
19th century.

● **INFLUENZA**
Gelsemium is used for
acute influenza. It eases
sore throats, limp limbs,
chills, fever (including
that accompanied by a
lack of thirst), headaches
with double vision, and
heavy, drooping eyelids.

● **HAY FEVER**
If accompanied by any of
the symptoms mentioned
under *Influenza*, hay fever
may be treated effectively
with *Gelsemium*.

GRAPHITES

Treats glandular disorders ◆ Soothes irritated, [...]

and infected skin ◆ Eases painful periods

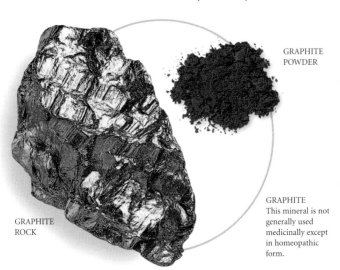

GRAPHITE
POWDER

GRAPHITE
This mineral is not
generally used
medicinally except
in homeopathic
form.

GRAPHITE
ROCK

KEY ACTIONS

- AIDS DIGESTION
- EASES PAINFUL BREASTS
- RELIEVES CONSTIPATION, BLOATING, AND FLATULENCE
- TREATS UROGENITARY DISORDERS

KEY PREPARATIONS

- TINCTURE made from graphite powder. It is triturated with lactose sugar to make it soluble. After being dissolved in water, it is repeatedly diluted and succussed.

INDICATIONS

● **ERECTILE PROBLEMS**
Graphites is effective for impotence in men with a high libido at an early age. It is also prescribed for priapism (persistent, sore erection).

● **MENSTRUATION**
Irregular, scanty periods and swollen, hard, painful breasts before and during menstruation can be eased with this remedy. It also treats itchy genitals and constipation during menstruation.

● **SKIN CONDITIONS**
Irritated skin, eczema, psoriasis, and cracked skin may be alleviated with *Graphites*. As may ill-

conditioned nails. The remedy is also effective for painful scars, cold sores, and genital herpes.

● **DIGESTIVE PROBLEMS**
Graphites is given for constipation, bloating, and flatulence. It is also effective for anal fissures, hemorrhoids, rectal itching, and stomach pains accompanied by hunger or vomiting.

● **GLANDS**
Graphites is commonly prescribed for physical symptoms that tend to affect the left side of the body and are often linked to glandular problems. Sensitivity to the cold and headaches after skipping meals are also typical.

HAMAMELIS

Treats varicose veins ◆ Relieves hemorrhoids

Useful first aid remedy

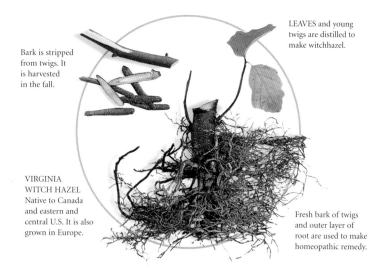

Bark is stripped from twigs. It is harvested in the fall.

LEAVES and young twigs are distilled to make witchhazel.

VIRGINIA WITCH HAZEL Native to Canada and eastern and central U.S. It is also grown in Europe.

Fresh bark of twigs and outer layer of root are used to make homeopathic remedy.

KEY ACTIONS

- EASES HEAVY PERIODS
- DISINFECTS
- EASES INFLAMMATION

KEY PREPARATIONS

- TINCTURE made from fresh chopped bark taken from the twigs and roots, steeped in alcohol.

INDICATIONS

● VARICOSE VEINS

This condition is caused when the valves inside the veins start to fail and blood pools form. They appear as twisted, purple lines, mainly affecting the legs. *Hamamelis* is prescribed for varicose veins with a sore, bruised feeling. Varicose veins may be hereditary, or may result from pregnancy, obesity, or thrombosis.

● HEMORRHOIDS

Hemorrhoids, also known as "piles," are swollen veins in the lower rectum and around the anus. They are often due to constipation, but also associated with hormonal problems, pregnancy, childbirth, the overuse of laxatives, and sitting on hard surfaces. *Hamamelis* is considered most effective for those type of hemorrhoids which, in appearance, resemble a bunch of grapes.

● FIRST AID

Hamamelis, also known as Virginia witch hazel, is valued as an herbal first aid remedy for its astringent properties.

● BLEEDING

This remedy is given to those with a susceptibility to hemorrhaging, such as women who suffer from heavy periods, or people who experience extreme nosebleeds.

HEPAR SULF.

Eases respiratory problems ◆ Heals skin infections

Treats digestive disorders

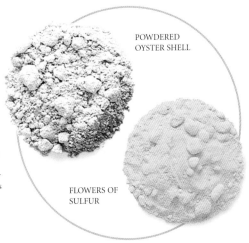

POWDERED OYSTER SHELL

Hepar sulf. is a form of calcium sulfide using powdered oyster shell and flowers of sulfur.

FLOWERS OF SULFUR

KEY ACTIONS

- REDUCES FEVER
- TREATS SWOLLEN GLANDS
- SOOTHES PAINFUL SKIN
- PROMOTES HEALING

KEY PREPARATIONS

- TINCTURE made from flowers of sulfur and powdered oyster shell. They are heated, dissolved in acid, and triturated with lactose sugar.

INDICATIONS

● **INFECTIONS**
Hepar sulf. is generally used where there is an infection, particularly in the respiratory system or the skin (such as styes, boils, and herpes). It is particularly appropriate for ailments that are accompanied by swollen glands, especially in the neck or groin, or if there is a high fever alternating with chills.

● **COUGHS & COLDS**
Colds or influenza with fever; sore throats with swollen tonsils; dry, hacking coughs; and croup are treated with *Hepar sulf.* It reduces the risk of a secondary

infection, loosens phlegm, and brings down fever.

● **SKIN CONDITIONS**
This remedy is prescribed for skin that chaps or roughens easily, or where inflamed, sore acne is present. It promotes healing in skin where eruptions are slow to heal and prone to infection.

● **ABSCESSES & ULCERS**
Hepar sulf. is given to treat abscesses or ulcers that bleed easily and are at risk of infection.

● **DIGESTION**
Use *Hepar sulf.* to treat nausea, vomiting, and chronic diarrhea accompanied by a grumbling abdomen.

MERC. SOL.

Cures halitosis ◆ Treats oral and genital thrush

Relieves the symptoms of osteoarthritis

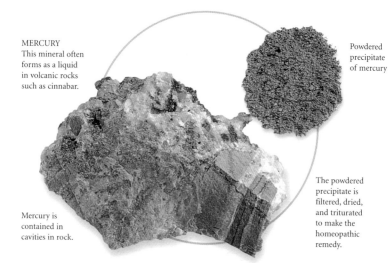

MERCURY
This mineral often
forms as a liquid
in volcanic rocks
such as cinnabar.

Powdered
precipitate
of mercury

The powdered
precipitate is
filtered, dried,
and triturated
to make the
homeopathic
remedy.

Mercury is
contained in
cavities in rock.

KEY ACTIONS

- FIGHTS INFECTION
- PAIN-RELIEVING
- SOOTHES MOUTH
  ULCERS AND ABSCESSES
- REDUCES FEVER

KEY PREPARATIONS

- POWDER made from
  mercury dissolved in
  nitric acid. This forms
  a gray powder
  precipitate which is
  filtered, dried, and
  triturated until
  soluble.

INDICATIONS

● **ARTHRITIS**
Merc. sol. is prescribed to
relieve osteoarthritis.

● **HALITOSIS**
Halitosis (bad breath) can
be caused by tooth decay,
smoking, gingivitis,
indigestion, tonsillitis,
sinusitis, or fasting.
Halitosis associated with
tooth decay and gingivitis
with bleeding gums, are
treated with *Merc. sol.*

● **MOUTH & THROAT
CONDITIONS**
Merc. sol. may be given
for mouth ulcers; sore,
raised, cream-colored
patches, usually indicative
of oral thrush; abscesses;
aching teeth caused by

bleeding or infected
gums; and sore throats.

● **YEAST INFECTION**
Merc. sol. treats yeast
infection.

● **INFECTION**
Eye and ear infections can
be alleviated by this
remedy, as can colds,
rhinitis, and fever.

● **CAUTION**
Non-homeopathic doses
of mercury were used as
an aggressive treatment
for syphilis and other
diseases. It was given to
Charles II and George
Washington. Its use
persisted to c. 1900 when
it was stopped, in the
West, its toxic effects
deemed too dangerous.

HYOSCYAMUS

Alleviates the early symptoms of Parkinson's disease

Aids stroke victims ◆ Treats paranoia

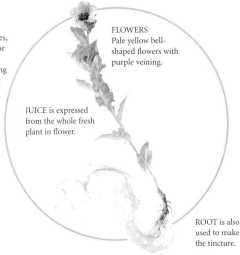

HENBANE
In the Middle Ages, the Latin name for henbane was *Dentaris*, signifying its use as a herbal remedy for toothache.

FLOWERS
Pale yellow bell-shaped flowers with purple veining.

JUICE is expressed from the whole fresh plant in flower.

ROOT is also used to make the tincture.

KEY ACTIONS

- RELAXES MUSCLES
- CALMS
- RELIEVES FEELINGS OF CONFUSION, JEALOUSY, AND PARANOIA

KEY PREPARATIONS

- TINCTURE made from the whole, fresh plant in flower, including the root. It is chopped finely, steeped in alcohol for 10 days, diluted, and succussed.

INDICATIONS

● **PARKINSON'S DISEASE**
The antispasmodic properties of *Hyoscyamus* (also known as henbane) are used by herbalists to relieve tremors and rigidity experienced during the early stages of Parkinson's disease.

● **STROKE**
Hyoscyamus is effective for treating a paralytic stroke that is associated with confused and inappropriate behavior.

● **PARANOIA**
This remedy is given to sufferers of severe paranoia and jealousy, suspicious of being watched, deceived, or even poisoned. This may be exacerbated by PMS or emotional stress.

● **ANESTHETIC**
The leaves are high in the sedative alkaloid hyoscine, used to make a conventional pre-operative anesthetic.

● **CAUTION**
The leaves may cause skin irritation on contact. Taken in non-homeopathic doses, henbane is highly poisonous: it was the method by which Shakespeare had Hamlet's father murdered, and infamous Dr. Crippen used it to murder his wife.

HYPERICUM

Relieves depression   ◆   Prevents tetanus

Treats phantom limb pain

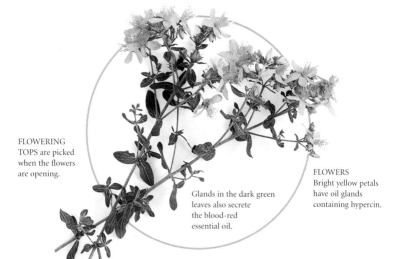

FLOWERING TOPS are picked when the flowers are opening.

Glands in the dark green leaves also secrete the blood-red essential oil.

FLOWERS
Bright yellow petals have oil glands containing hypercin.

KEY ACTIONS

- RELIEVES PAIN
- CALMS
- CURES TOOTHACHE

KEY PREPARATIONS

- TINCTURE made from the whole, fresh plant. It is finely chopped and macerated in alcohol.

INDICATIONS

● **DEPRESSION**
Hypericum perf., also known as St. John's wort, has been renowned since classical times. It is given to those who are shocked, frightened, or depressed. Those who benefit from it may be overexcited, nervous, continually drowsy, or forgetful. They may also experience a constant sensation of elevation or falling.

● **INJURIES**
Key physical symptoms associated with this remedy are injuries and wounds that feel more painful than they appear, with occurrences of extremely sharp pains,

perhaps in nerve-rich areas, such as the fingertips or the base of the spine. It may be used to relieve pain following operations, accidents, or puncture wounds.

● **ANIMAL BITES**
St. John's wort may be administered to a patient who has been bitten by an animal to help prevent tetanus.

● **PHANTOM LIMB PAIN**
The remedy is effective in treating pains experienced after amputation.

● **DENTAL CARE**
St. John's wort is given to cure toothache. It is also used to relieve pain after dental surgery.

IGNATIA

Eases acute grief

Relieves emotional stress ◆ Treats insomnia

IGNATIA SEEDS
These seeds are very
bitter, due to the
poisonous
strychnine they
contain.

SEED PODS
Each seed pod
contains about
10 to 20 seeds.

The plant is native
to the East Indies,
China, and the
Phillipine Islands.

The seeds are separated
from the pulp and
powdered to make the
homeopathic remedy.

KEY ACTIONS

- CALMS
- AIDS WITH THE GRIEVING PROCESS
- PROMOTES GOOD DIGESTION
- TREATS MENSTRUAL PROBLEMS

KEY PREPARATIONS

- TINCTURE made from the dried seeds. They are powdered before being steeped in alcohol for at least five days. This is followed by filtration, dilution, and succussion.

INDICATIONS

● GRIEF
Ignatia is used to treat the initial impact of grief. It is particularly effective for women and is often given after a bereavement or the break-up of a relationship. Follow-up remedies may then be prescribed.

● AMENORRHEA
Amenorrhea is the absence of menstruation. Homeopaths may prescribe *Ignatia* when periods stop as a result of emotional stress.

● STRESS
The remedy is effective in treating illness that develops from emotional stress (*see above*). This

includes headaches; nervous tics and twitches; digestive disorders, such as nausea and vomiting; and a sore throat.

● HICCUPS
Hiccups associated with emotional stress are treated with *Ignatia*.

● INSOMNIA
Insomnia has several causes and effects. This remedy is prescribed for insomnia accompanied by a fear of never being able to fall asleep again.

● CAUTION
The seeds contain strychnine, a poison that acts on the nervous system when taken in non-homeopathic doses.

KALI. BICH.

Soothes mucous membranes

Eases respiratory trouble ◆ Treats rheumatoid arthritis

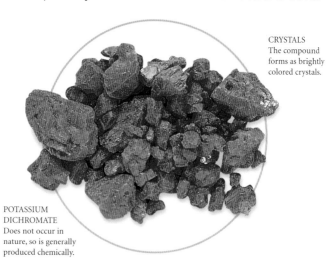

CRYSTALS
The compound forms as brightly colored crystals.

POTASSIUM DICHROMATE
Does not occur in nature, so is generally produced chemically.

KEY ACTIONS

- EASES INFLAMMATION
- PROMOTES SKIN HEALING
- FIGHTS INFECTION
- RELIEVES PAIN

KEY PREPARATIONS

- TINCTURE made from crystals of potassium dichromate. These are triturated with lactose sugar until soluble in water. They are then filtered, diluted, and succussed.

INDICATIONS

● **ARTHRITIS**
Kali. bich. is prescribed for rheumatoid arthritis and other types of joint pain.

● **SINUSITIS**
Sinusitis occurs when the mucous membranes lining the sinuses become inflamed, due to allergy or infection. This remedy is effective for sinusitis with stringy mucus.

● **GLUE EAR**
A condition resulting from overactivity of the mucous membrane lining the middle ear, or caused by allergy. A buildup of sticky fluid leads to reduced hearing. If it is accompanied by thick, stringy mucus, *Kali. bich.* may be prescribed.

● **BREATHING TROUBLE**
As *Kali. bich.* is considered beneficial for the mucous membranes (*see above*), it is given for respiratory-tract ailments, especially with excessive mucus.

● **SKIN CONDITIONS**
The remedy is used to heal ulcers, acne, and other skin conditions accompanied by discharge or burning pain.

● **CAUTION**
Potassium dichromate, the compound used to make this remedy, is highly caustic and poisonous in non-homeopathic doses.

KALI. CARB.

Treats kidney disorders ◆ Treats whooping cough and other chest infections ◆ Relieves insomnia

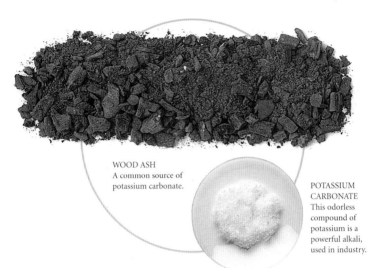

WOOD ASH
A common source of potassium carbonate.

POTASSIUM CARBONATE
This odorless compound of potassium is a powerful alkali, used in industry.

KEY ACTIONS

- RELIEVES PAIN
- EASES INFLAMMATION
- RELIEVES INSOMNIA
- CALMS
- EASES OSTEOARTHRITIS

KEY PREPARATIONS

- TINCTURE made from potassium carbonate triturated with lactose sugar until it is soluble in water. This solution is then diluted and succussed.

INDICATIONS

● **PAIN RELIEF**
This remedy is associated with pain in the joints, back, or kidneys.

● **COUGHS & COLDS**
Dry, hacking, expectorant coughs, whooping cough, or wheezy coughs, may all be treated with *Kali. carb.*

● **INSOMNIA**
Insomnia with difficulty falling asleep, or getting to sleep but waking again, is treated with *Kali. carb.*

● **ASTHMA**
Kali. carb. is prescribed for patients who regularly suffer asthma attacks between 2 and 4 A.M., causing exhaustion.

● **ARTHRITIS**
Kali. carb. is one of several remedies indicated for osteoarthritis.

● **PALPITATIONS**
It is given for palpitations that are accompanied by respiratory problems.

● **KIDNEY DISORDERS**
Kidney stones or other diseases of the kidney are treated with this remedy, especially those with shooting pains in the small of the back. The pains may be worse on the left side.

● **CAUTION**
Non-homeopathic doses are rarely prescribed due to its highly caustic nature.

KALI. MUR.

Treats chronic rhinitis ◆ Helps heal nasal

and aural problems ◆ Eases inflamed joints

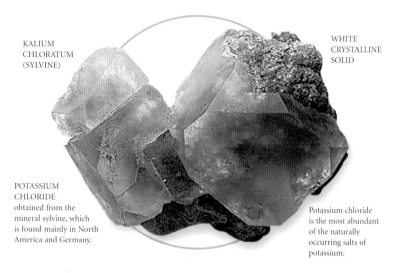

KALIUM
CHLORATUM
(SYLVINE)

WHITE
CRYSTALLINE
SOLID

POTASSIUM
CHLORIDE
obtained from the
mineral sylvine, which
is found mainly in North
America and Germany.

Potassium chloride
is the most abundant
of the naturally
occurring salts of
potassium.

KEY ACTIONS

- EASES INFLAMMATION
- RELIEVES CONGESTION
- RELIEVES PAIN

KEY PREPARATIONS

- TINCTURE made from powdered potassium chloride triturated with lactose sugar.

INDICATIONS

● **CANCER**
Kali. mur. is indicated in the treatment for cancer of the connective tissue and of the throat.

● **NASAL PROBLEMS**
Congestion of the nose, due to profuse, whitish mucus, and with the presence of nosebleeds, is treated with *Kali. mur.*

● **EARS**
The remedy is particularly effective for the middle ear, with accompanying earache, pain behind the ears, snapping noises, blockage of the eustachian tube (especially if accompanied by mucus), and possible deafness.

● **TONSILITIS**
Kali. mur. is an important remedy for tonsilitis or swollen throat glands. It is also used for chronic sore throats with crusts of mucus in the throat.

● **INFLAMMATION**
Kali. mur. is effective in reducing inflammation; it is most usually prescribed to treat inflamed membranes or joints.

● **EMOTIONS**
People who respond best to *Kali. mur.* tend to be optimistic and hard working, but also tend to alternate between cheerfulness and sadness, being sensitive to sadness in others as well as in themselves.

KREOSOTUM

Treats menstrual problems

Heals mucus membranes ◆ Soothes candidiasis

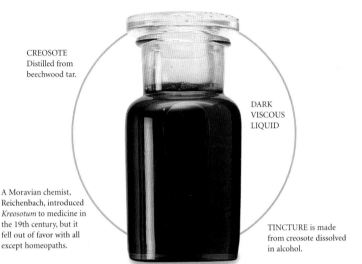

CREOSOTE
Distilled from
beechwood tar.

DARK
VISCOUS
LIQUID

A Moravian chemist,
Reichenbach, introduced
Kreosotum to medicine in
the 19th century, but it
fell out of favor with all
except homeopaths.

TINCTURE is made
from creosote dissolved
in alcohol.

KEY ACTIONS

- EASES INFLAMMATION
- SOOTHES
- TREATS CERTAIN
  EMOTIONAL PROBLEMS
- PROMOTES GOOD
  HEALTH IN WOMEN

KEY PREPARATIONS

- TINCTURE made from
  creosote dissolved in
  alcohol, diluted, and
  succussed.

INDICATIONS

● **MUCUS MEMBRANES**
The classic symptom
picture associated with
Kreosotum is of mucus
membranes that become
inflamed, suppurate, and
break down and bleed,
particularly in the vagina,
cervix, and the uterus.

● **CANDIDIASIS**
This is one of several
remedies that may be
prescribed for candidiasis
(yeast overgrowth).

● **EMOTIONS & PHOBIAS**
People who respond best
to *Kreosotum* may be
temperamental, forgetful,
peevish, sensitive to
music, or restless at night.
A tendency to dwell on

the past, dreams of sexual
intercourse, and a fear of
being raped are typical.

● **DISCHARGE**
The remedy is given for
offensive-smelling
discharges from the
mucus membranes that
burn the skin and cause
itching and swelling. It
may also help with
conditions where urine
burns the skin on contact.

● **MENSTRUATION**
It may be prescribed for
particular problems
associated with
menstruation, such as
bleeding between usual
cycles and heavy,
offensive-smelling
menstrual flow that burns
the skin on contact.

LACHESIS

Calms hot flashes ◆ Treats circulatory problems

Relieves spasms and tremors

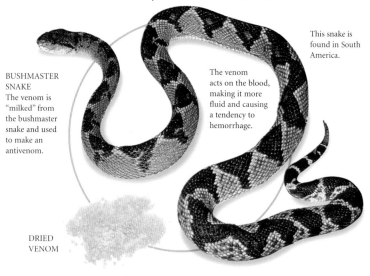

This snake is found in South America.

BUSHMASTER SNAKE
The venom is "milked" from the bushmaster snake and used to make an antivenom.

The venom acts on the blood, making it more fluid and causing a tendency to hemorrhage.

DRIED VENOM

KEY ACTIONS

- DEALS WITH LEFT-SIDED SYMPTOMS
- SOOTHES ANXIETY
- RELIEVES PAIN
- CALMS MUSCLE SPASMS

KEY PREPARATIONS

- TINCTURE made from venom "milked" from the bushmaster snake before being dissolved in alcohol. The mixture is then repeatedly diluted and succussed.

INDICATIONS

● **HOT FLASHES**
Lachesis calms hot flashes that occur during the menopause, premenstrual syndrome, and certain nervous disorders.

● **ENERGY**
People who respond well to this remedy have fluctuating energy levels. When ill, symptoms may develop on the left side and develop or worsen during sleep.

● **CIRCULATION**
Poor circulation that turns the face, ears, and extremities blue or purple can be treated with *Lachesis*. It is prescribed for wounds that bleed

easily, and for engorged, bluish-purple varicose veins. It also treats cramping chest pains.

● **WOMEN'S HEALTH**
In addition to treating hot flushes (*see above*), *Lachesis* is effective for painful menstruation, perhaps with fainting spells, hot sweats, and left-sided headaches or violent mood swings that occur premenstrually.

● **SPASMS & TREMORS**
Lachesis is given for muscle spasms, tremors, and weakness in the limbs, possibly linked to alcoholism, multiple sclerosis, fever, petit mal epilepsy, or brain damage after a stroke.

LEDUM

Eases painful joints and arthritic pain

Heals cuts and wounds ◆ Treats painful eye problems

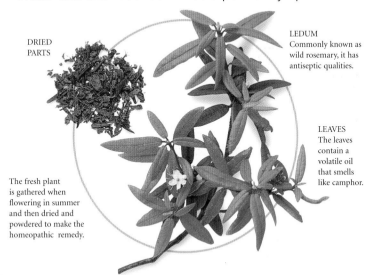

DRIED PARTS

LEDUM
Commonly known as wild rosemary, it has antiseptic qualities.

LEAVES
The leaves contain a volatile oil that smells like camphor.

The fresh plant is gathered when flowering in summer and then dried and powdered to make the homeopathic remedy.

KEY ACTIONS

- DISINFECTANT
- SLOWS BLEEDING
- EASES INFLAMMATION

KEY PREPARATIONS

- TINCTURE made from the tips of the leafy shoots. They are collected as the plant comes into flower, then dried and steeped in alcohol.

INDICATIONS

● **FIRST AID**
This remedy is also known as marsh tea and wild rosemary. For years it has been considered a key first aid treatment for cuts, grazes, puncture wounds, insect stings, and black eyes.

● **PAINFUL JOINTS**
Rheumatic pains that start in the feet and move up are relieved by *Ledum*, as are stiff, painful joints that feel hot inside despite being cold to the touch. For osteoarthritis sufferers, the remedy is given for joints that feel cold, are swollen, and make cracking noises on moving. If a joint complaint is relieved by cold compresses, it will respond well to *Ledum*.

● **EYE CONDITIONS**
In addition to treating black eyes (*see left*), especially those slow to heal, *Ledum* treats other eye injuries including stemming bleeding in the eye after an iridectomy (the removal of part of the iris).

● **INFECTION**
Ledum prevents infection in open wounds, such as severe wounds with bruised, puffy, purplish skin and stinging pains. Its disinfectant properties led to its traditional use in Scandinavia: to eliminate body lice.

LILIUM

Treats angina and other heart disorders

Used for women's health problems ◆ Relieves depression

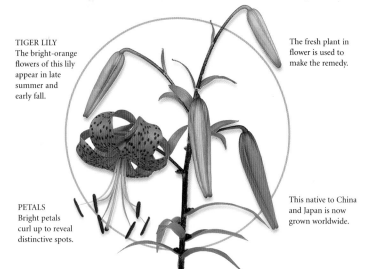

TIGER LILY
The bright-orange flowers of this lily appear in late summer and early fall.

The fresh plant in flower is used to make the remedy.

PETALS
Bright petals curl up to reveal distinctive spots.

This native to China and Japan is now grown worldwide.

KEY ACTIONS

- TREATS URINARY DISORDERS
- SOOTHES ANXIETY
- RELIEVES PAIN
- UPLIFTS EMOTIONS

KEY PREPARATIONS

- TINCTURE made from the stalk, leaves, and flowers of the fresh plant. They are chopped finely and soaked in alcohol for at least 10 days. The mixture is then filtered, diluted, and succussed.

INDICATIONS

● **URINARY DISORDERS**
Cystitis (usually in women) with burning, stinging pain during and after urination is treated with this remedy. It helps to reduce the patient's constant need to pass urine when only a small amount is being passed at any one time.

● **WOMEN'S HEALTH**
Disorders of the female reproductive system, such as uterine prolapse, vulval itching, and a bearing-down pain in the pelvis, may be treated with *Lilium*. Fibroids may also be treated with the remedy, and it may be recommended for swollen ovaries or painful menstruation.

● **DEPRESSION**
A sense of despair and a need for religious salvation is characteristic in people who need *Lilium*. They may have a fear of developing an incurable disease and look for a reason to grieve.

● **ANGINA**
Lilium is prescribed when the chest feels as though it is being gripped in a vise, and there are palpitations and pain in the right arm. It is also given for other heart disorders, such as rapid or irregular pulse, poor circulation, or palpitations that occur during pregnancy.

LYCOPODIUM

Treats urogenitary and prostate disorders

Eases anxiety ◆ Alleviates digestive problems

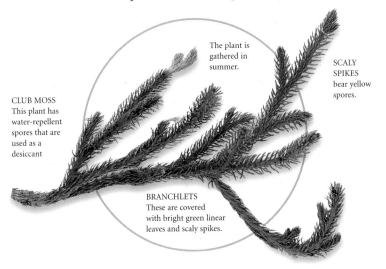

The plant is gathered in summer.

SCALY SPIKES bear yellow spores.

CLUB MOSS This plant has water-repellent spores that are used as a desiccant

BRANCHLETS These are covered with bright green linear leaves and scaly spikes.

KEY ACTIONS

- KILLS BACTERIA
- CALMS ANXIETY
- FIGHTS INFECTION

KEY PREPARATIONS

- TINCTURE made from the spikes of Lycopodium. They are cut in summer, and their spores are collected. They are then steeped in alcohol for at least five days before being filtered, diluted, and succussed.

INDICATIONS

● **PROSTATE PROBLEMS**
Lycopodium is one of several homeopathic remedies recommended for prostate disorders. It is prescribed when the prostate has become enlarged. It is also given to treat urine with a sandy sediment due to kidney stones, and for genital herpes. *Lycopodium* was used in the 17th century to ease urine retention.

● **ANXIETY**
Traditionally used for its sedative action, this remedy is prescribed to those who suffer from insomnia, talking and laughing while asleep, night fears, and apprehension upon waking. Anticipatory anxiety, such as fear of public speaking, exams, or performing onstage, all of which often lead to digestive disorders, are treated with *Lycopodium*.

● **DIGESTIVE DISORDER**
This remedy is given for indigestion, such as that caused by anticipatory anxiety (*see above*); nausea; vomiting; constipation; and also bleeding hemorrhoids.

● **CHEST INFECTIONS**
Dry, sore, tickling coughs; burning chest pains; and fast, labored breathing can be eased with *Lycopodium*; as can sore throats and severe rhinitis.

MAG. PHOS.

Treats neuralgia ◆ Eases abdominal pains and other cramps

Relieves headaches, toothache, and earache

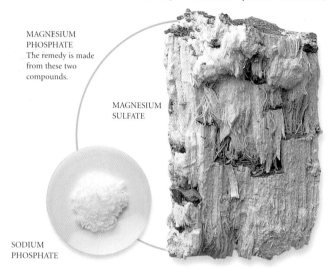

MAGNESIUM
PHOSPHATE
The remedy is made
from these two
compounds.

MAGNESIUM
SULFATE

SODIUM
PHOSPHATE

KEY ACTIONS

- RELIEVES PAIN
- CALMS SPASMS
- DEALS CHIEFLY WITH RIGHT-SIDED PAIN
- SOOTHES MENSTRUAL CRAMPS
- RELIEVES IRRITABLE BOWEL SYNDROME

KEY PREPARATIONS

- TINCTURE made from magnesium sulfate and sodium phosphate mixed in water and left to crystallize. The resulting crystals are then triturated with lactose sugar.

INDICATIONS

● **MENSTRUAL CRAMPS**
Taken for sudden cramping, shooting pains in the lower abdomen during menstruation. Also given for nonmenstrual abdominal cramps, such as those associated with irritable bowel syndrome.

● **EARACHE**
The remedy relieves pains in the ear that are spasmodic and shooting, especially following exposure to cold wind.

● **TOOTHACHE**
Dull, throbbing pain or sharp twinges of pain, especially common in teething infants, can be treated with *Mag. phos.*

● **NEURALGIA**
Mag. phos. is prescribed for sharp, radiating, cramping pains that appear and disappear rapidly anywhere in the body. It relieves muscles that are stiff, numb, and awkward, especially after exertion.

● **HEADACHE**
Given for spasmodic, shooting pains on the right side, or back of the neck; pains that spread over the head and settle around the right eye.

● **CRAMPS**
Treats sudden onset of cramps in the fingers, arms, wrists, and hands, common in musicians and writers.

NAT. MUR.

Treats women's health disorders ◆ Promotes good digestion

Relieves migraines and headaches

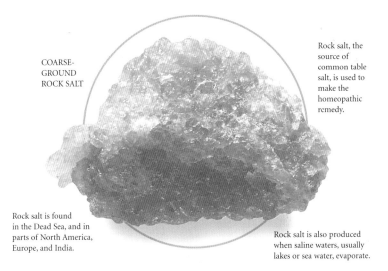

COARSE-
GROUND
ROCK SALT

Rock salt, the source of common table salt, is used to make the homeopathic remedy.

Rock salt is found in the Dead Sea, and in parts of North America, Europe, and India.

Rock salt is also produced when saline waters, usually lakes or sea water, evaporate.

KEY ACTIONS

- HEALS MOUTH ULCERS, ABSCESSES, AND GINGIVITIS
- EASES MENSTRUAL PROBLEMS
- SOOTHES SKIN CONDITIONS

KEY PREPARATIONS

- TINCTURE made from rock salt dissolved in boiling water, filtered, and evaporated to make pure sodium chloride. This is then triturated with lactose sugar. Historically, salt had economic value, but has had limited medicinal uses outside homeopathy.

INDICATIONS

● **HEADACHES**
The remedy relieves hammering, bursting headaches and migraines that occur above the eyes. It also treats those headaches and migraines accompanied by vision distortion, such as zigzag lines.

● **DIGESTION**
Nat. mur. is prescribed for constipation where the stools are dry and hard, causing colicky pains with nausea, backache, and possible anal bleeding.

● **WOMEN'S HEALTH**
Used to cure fatigue, water retention, and severe headaches occurring around menstruation. Also given to treat white vaginal discharge, usually due to yeast infection. Has been effective in treating vaginismus, where painful spasms occur during intercourse, and for patients whose periods have stopped due to grief or shock.

● **SKIN CONDITIONS**
Greasy skin and hair, dandruff, warts, boils, psoriasis, urticaria (hives), hangnails, and facial herpes may be helped by the remedy.

● **MOUTH & THROAT**
Nat. mur. heals mouth ulcers, dental abscesses, gingivitis (bleeding gums), and cracked lips.

NAT. SULF.

Eases liver problems ◆ Treats headaches

Relieves asthma

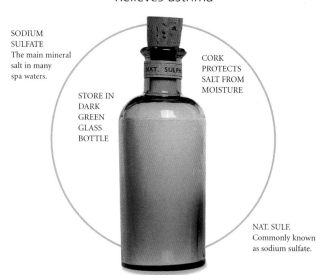

SODIUM SULFATE
The main mineral salt in many spa waters.

CORK PROTECTS SALT FROM MOISTURE

STORE IN DARK GREEN GLASS BOTTLE

NAT. SULPH

NAT. SULF.
Commonly known as sodium sulfate.

KEY ACTIONS

- PROMOTES GOOD DIGESTION
- TREATS DEPRESSION
- SOOTHES HEADACHES
- TREATS HEPATITIS
- EASES GALLSTONES

KEY PREPARATIONS

- TINCTURE made from sodium sulfate triturated with lactose sugar.

INDICATIONS

● **HEADACHES**
Nat. sulf. has an affinity with head symptoms, such as headaches due to injury, or those accompanied by increased salivation or strong intolerance to light.

● **DEPRESSION**
The remedy is prescribed for severe or suicidal depression, and for profound mental changes, possibly with suicidal thoughts, following a head injury.

● **EMOTIONS**
Nat. sulf. is best suited to people who are serious, reserved, responsible, and focused on work, yet paradoxically highly sensitive; music may move them to tears. They may feel isolated from intimate, committed relationships, perhaps after losing a partner.

● **ASTHMA**
This is a major remedy for asthma brought on by damp conditions.

● **LIVER PROBLEMS**
Problems with the liver, the digestive system, gallbladder, pancreas, and spleen may be treated with *Nat. sulf.* Liver conditions treated by the remedy include hepatitis and gallstones with bitter belching, colicky abdominal pains, and jaundice.

OPIUM

Alleviates insomnia ◆ Helps with post-stroke treatment

Treats shock

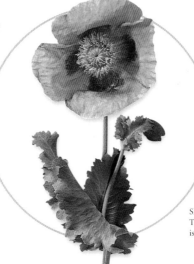

OPIUM POPPY
Flowers appear in late summer and early fall.

Native to western Asia, opium poppy is now cultivated commercially around the world.

DULL GREEN LEAVES AND THICK STEM

SEED CAPSULES
These contain a latex that is the source of morphine.

KEY ACTIONS

- RELIEVES CONSTIPATION
- TREATS DELIRIUM TREMENS
- HELPS WITH NARCOLEPSY
- AIDS ALCOHOL WITHDRAWAL

KEY PREPARATIONS

- TINCTURE made from the sap of the unripe green seed pods, dried, dissolved in alcohol, and succussed.

INDICATIONS

● **DELIRIUM TREMENS**
Extreme apathy or hypersensitivity, tremors, or convulsions resulting from delirium tremens are treated with *Opium*. It is also prescribed to aid with alcohol withdrawal.

● **SHOCK & INJURY**
Emotional responses to shock, grief, or injury can be treated with *Opium*, as can physical responses, such as convulsions.

● **INSOMNIA**
Opium has been used as a sedative and analgesic since antiquity. It was dedicated by the Greeks and Romans to the gods of night, death, and dreams. Insomnia, an inability to sleep despite fatigue, and brief bouts of irresistible drowsiness can be treated with *Opium*. It is also indicated for the treatment of narcolepsy.

● **CONSTIPATION**
Newborn babies may be given *Opium* to relieve constipation after the shock of birth. Children and adults are also treated with the remedy.

● **POST-STROKE CARE**
The remedy treats paralysis of the limbs with dullness and stupor resembling that experienced after shock, possibly with blackouts. It is also used for resultant brain injuries.

PHOSPHORUS

Stems heavy bleeding ◆ Helps with poor circulation

Treats respiratory problems

PHOSPHORUS
This yellowish-white solid glows in the dark and is highly flammable.

PHOSPHORUS REMEDY

Phosphorus is kept under water because it catches fire spontaneously on exposure to air.

Profuse bleeding from the gums is one of the conditions helped by this remedy.

KEY ACTIONS

- TREATS ASTHMA, BRONCHITIS, AND PNEUMONIA
- IMPROVES CIRCULATION
- PROMOTES GOOD DIGESTION

KEY PREPARATIONS

- TINCTURE made from white phosphorus. This waxy substance is insoluble in water, so it is dissolved in alcohol, filtered, then repeatedly diluted and succussed.

INDICATIONS

● **DIGESTIVE PROBLEMS**
Phosphorus is given for digestive disorders where the stools are streaked with blood. It may be prescribed for stomach ulcers, gastroenteritis, food poisoning, and stomach trouble caused by stress.

● **BLEEDING**
Profuse bleeding, from the nose, gums, and stomach lining, is treated with *Phosphorus*. It is also given for heavy menstrual flow.

● **POOR CIRCULATION**
Given to reduce the effects of poor circulation, including erratic blood flow causing hot flashes;

palpitations; and fainting, characterized by a weak pulse. Treats extremities that feel burning hot yet are cold to the touch.

● **RESPIRATORY ILLNESS**
The remedy is used for respiratory problems linked to anxiety and is associated with chest tightness due to asthma, bronchitis, or pneumonia. Symptoms treated may include phlegm streaked with dark-red blood, a sore throat, dry tickly cough, and possible retching or vomiting.

● **CAUTION**
This is highly toxic and should not be handled in its non-homeopathic form.

PHYTOLACCA

Eases breast problems ◆ Heals psoriasis

Treats glandular fever and other glandular disorders

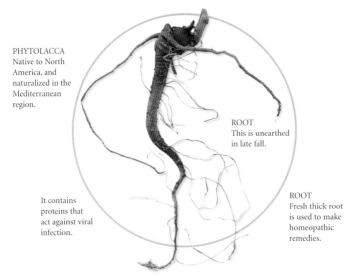

PHYTOLACCA
Native to North
America, and
naturalized in the
Mediterranean
region.

ROOT
This is unearthed
in late fall.

It contains
proteins that
act against viral
infection.

ROOT
Fresh thick root
is used to make
homeopathic
remedies.

KEY ACTIONS

- EASES INFLAMMATION
- RELIEVES PAIN
- TREATS MUMPS
- EASES DIFFICULT
  BREATHING

KEY PREPARATIONS

- TINCTURE made from
  the fresh root,
  unearthed during
  the fall. It is finely
  chopped and
  macerated in alcohol.

INDICATIONS

● **BREAST PROBLEMS**
Prescribed to treat cysts
that are tender before and
during menstruation. It is
also given for breast ulcers
and sometimes for breast
cancer. *Phytolacca* treats
mastitis with hardness,
burning, and pain in the
breasts that radiates
through the whole body
on breastfeeding.

● **PSORIASIS**
Phytolacca is prescribed to
sufferers of psoriasis when
there are lesions with a
purple coloration present.

● **GLANDS**
This remedy has a strong
affinity with the glands
and is used to treat

glandular fever. It is given
for hard, inflamed neck
glands, where pain in the
throat is present upon
swallowing. Inflamed
parotid glands, for
example during mumps,
may be helped by the
remedy. Also given for
inflamed, painful tonsils,
which may appear dark
red in color.

● **BREATHING**
When breathing feels
difficult, restricted, and
oppressed, with a sense of
suffocation and emptiness
in the chest, *Phytolacca*
may be prescribed.

● **CAUTION**
This plant is potent
and toxic if taken in
non-homeopathic form.

PULSATILLA

Heals eye infections ◆ Remedies

gynecological problems ◆ Relieves sinusitis

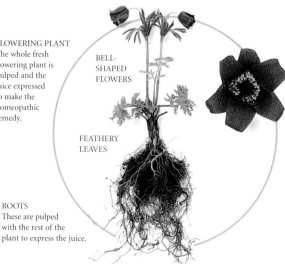

FLOWERING PLANT
The whole fresh flowering plant is pulped and the juice expressed to make the homeopathic remedy.

BELL-SHAPED FLOWERS

FLOWERS
The plant is distinguished from other *Pulsatilla* species by its smaller, purplish-black flowerheads.

FEATHERY LEAVES

ROOTS
These are pulped with the rest of the plant to express the juice.

KEY ACTIONS

- REDUCES FEVER
- PROMOTES GOOD DIGESTION
- EASES COUGHS AND COLDS
- TREATS INFLUENZA
- HELPS WITH PRE-MENSTRUAL SYNDROME

KEY PREPARATIONS

- TINCTURE made from the fresh flowering plant, including the root. It is chopped and macerated in alcohol, before being diluted and succussed.

INDICATIONS

● **EYE INFECTIONS**
Roman legend says this plant sprang from the tears of Venus, and was hence used for weepiness. *Pulsatilla* may help itchy eyes and conjunctivitis. In the 1st century A.D., Dioscorides, the Greek physician, prescribed it for eye problems.

● **WOMEN'S HEALTH**
Given for short, variable, late, or absent periods, and for severe menstrual pain. PMS may also respond to the remedy, and it is sometimes given to pregnant women, if the symptom picture fits. It can also be used to act on the uterine muscles and help turn a breech baby during labor.

● **SINUSITIS**
Pulsatilla is given when the sinuses are tender to the touch, with sharp pains beginning on the right side of the face, but tending to move around.

● **COUGHS & COLDS**
Treats wet, spasmodic coughing, with shortness of breath, worse for lying on the left side. *Pulsatilla* may also be prescribed for influenza with fever.

● **DIGESTIVE PROBLEMS**
Used for varied problems, including vomiting, nausea, indigestion, diarrhea, and painful, itchy hemorrhoids.

Rhus tox.

Eases musculoskeletal pain ◆ Heals infected skin

Soothes other painful skin complaints

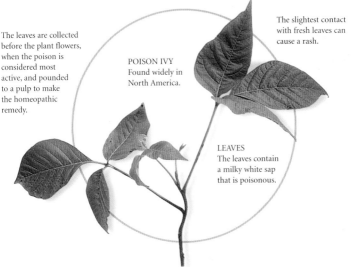

The leaves are collected before the plant flowers, when the poison is considered most active, and pounded to a pulp to make the homeopathic remedy.

POISON IVY
Found widely in
North America.

The slightest contact with fresh leaves can cause a rash.

LEAVES
The leaves contain a milky white sap that is poisonous.

KEY ACTIONS

- EASES INFLAMMATION
- FIGHTS INFECTIONS
- EASES ARTHRITIC PAIN
- TREATS ECZEMA AND OTHER SKIN PROBLEMS

KEY PREPARATIONS

- TINCTURE made from the fresh leaves, gathered at sunset just before the plant comes into flower. These are macerated in alcohol.

INDICATIONS

● JOINTS
Musculoskeletal problems are associated with *Rhus tox.*, and this remedy has become associated specifically with the joints. It is used to ease acute arthritis – both osteo- and rheumatoid – as well as sciatica, restless legs, cramps, and sprains.

● SKIN INFECTIONS
In addition to joint problems (*see above*), *Rhus tox.* is associated primarily with infection of the skin. It is effective for eczema and for conditions such as rosacea, where boils start to form. Infected eczema may start to ooze. The condition may be an allergic reaction, but the cause is often unknown. Childhood eczema usually clears up by adolescent puberty.

● SKIN CONDITIONS
Native Americans used this plant to treat skin eruptions and nervous paralysis. It may be helpful for skin eruptions with blisters, followed by burning, red, swollen skin that tends to scale and flake off. The remedy is given to treat chickenpox, shingles, herpes, and diaper rash.

● CAUTION
Contact with the plant's leaves produces redness, swelling, and blistering.

Ruta

Relieves eyestrain ◆ Eases muscular problems

Alleviates painful joints

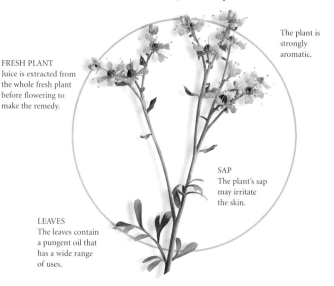

The plant is strongly aromatic.

FRESH PLANT
Juice is extracted from the whole fresh plant before flowering to make the remedy.

SAP
The plant's sap may irritate the skin.

LEAVES
The leaves contain a pungent oil that has a wide range of uses.

KEY ACTIONS

- CALMS
- RELIEVES PAIN
- HEALS STRAINED MUSCLES
- RELIEVES STIFFNESS IN MUSCLES AND JOINTS

KEY PREPARATIONS

- TINCTURE made from the aerial parts, gathered as the plant is beginning to flower. They are finely chopped and steeped in alcohol.

INDICATIONS

● **MENSTRUATION**
Ruta (also known as "Rue" or "herb-of-grace") has been prescribed herbally since the times of ancient Egypt and Greece to induce abortion and stimulate menstruation. The remedy may be given for menstrual problems.

● **MUSCLE PROBLEMS**
The classic symptom picture for *Ruta* is of connective tissue problems with marked stiffness and pain in the muscles and tendons, often due to sprains, overuse of the muscles, or injury. The pain is typically sore, bruised, aching, and accompanied by restlessness. The remedy is prescribed for repetitive strain injury.

● **EYE TREATMENTS**
Ruta is used to treat eyestrain (when the muscles have become weak), where burning pain is experienced. In ancient times the plant was used medicinally to strengthen eyesight.

● **JOINT PROBLEMS**
Used to treat chronic arthritis; a stiff, sore lower back; and sciatica.

● **EMOTIONS**
Those who respond best to the *Ruta* remedy are prone to feelings of anxiety and panic and tend to be weepy.

SEPIA

Treats women's health problems ◆ Soothes painful skin conditions ◆ Improves circulation

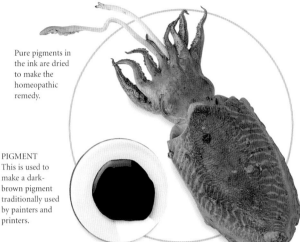

Pure pigments in the ink are dried to make the homeopathic remedy.

This soft mollusk is related to the octopus and squid. It squirts brownish-black ink for protection.

PIGMENT
This is used to make a dark-brown pigment traditionally used by painters and printers.

KEY ACTIONS

- RELIEVES PAIN
- SOOTHES
- CORRECTS HORMONAL IMBALANCE
- AIDS DIGESTION

KEY PREPARATIONS

- TINCTURE made from cuttlefish ink dried to a crystalline form and then triturated with lactose sugar.

INDICATIONS

● **WOMEN'S HEALTH**
Sepia, or cuttlefish ink, is predominantly prescribed to treat women's health problems, including hormone imbalances, especially those that occur before or during menstruation, or throughout menopause. It is also prescribed for some pregnancy-related ailments and can be used to treat yeast infection.

● **DIGESTIVE PROBLEMS**
Helps relieve indigestion, flatulence, vomiting, nausea, and constipation.

● **SKIN CONDITIONS**
The remedy is prescribed for itchy or discolored skin and a condition known as chloasma in which a yellowybrown "saddle" appears across the nose and cheeks, especially during pregnancy.

● **CIRCULATION**
The sepia remedy is given to help treat palpitations, varicose veins, and hot and cold flashes.

● **PAIN RELIEF**
Treats headaches that are prevalent on the left side, possibly with dizziness and nausea. Also relieves painful rhinitis, and signs of emotional and physical exhaustion, especially those accompanied by an aching back and sides and muscles that feel weak.

SILICA

Strengthens bones, teeth, hair, and nails

Promotes skin healing ◆ Treats food intolerances

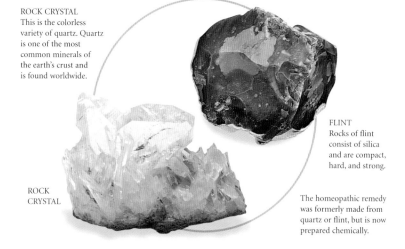

ROCK CRYSTAL
This is the colorless variety of quartz. Quartz is one of the most common minerals of the earth's crust and is found worldwide.

ROCK CRYSTAL

FLINT
Rocks of flint consist of silica and are compact, hard, and strong.

The homeopathic remedy was formerly made from quartz or flint, but is now prepared chemically.

KEY ACTIONS

- HEALS WOUNDS
- STRENGTHENS BONES
- SOOTHES
- RELIEVES PAIN
- FIGHTS INFECTION
- REMOVES FOREIGN BODIES FROM THE SKIN

KEY PREPARATIONS

- TINCTURE made by triturating silicon dioxide, grinding the sand repeatedly with lactose sugar until it becomes soluble in water, then diluting and succussing it.

INDICATIONS

● BONES & TEETH
Silica promotes healing in brittle bones, and is given for curvature of the spine. It is used for slow-healing problems and to improve children's health, such as fontanelles that close slowly. It is given for slow eruption of teeth and to ease wisdom tooth pain.

● SKIN, HAIR, & NAILS
The remedy heals defects due to poor absorption of minerals in the diet. It heals brittle, distorted, infected nails and ingrown toenails. It is used to encourage healing in wounds that suppurate and heal slowly, abscesses, itchy scars, and acne.

● REMOVING SPLINTERS
Silica has the unusual feature of being able to help expel foreign bodies such as splinters from the skin.

● HEADACHES
Severe pain starting at the back of the head and extending over to the forehead, with dizziness and visual disturbances, is treated with *Silica*.

● DIGESTIVE PROBLEMS
Prescribed for a weak digestive system, with food intolerances.

● COUGHS & COLDS
Silica is used for persistent or recurrent coughs, colds, and infections of the ear, nose, and throat.

DULCAMARA

Eases painful joints ◆ Treats hay fever and asthma
Relieves head and facial pain

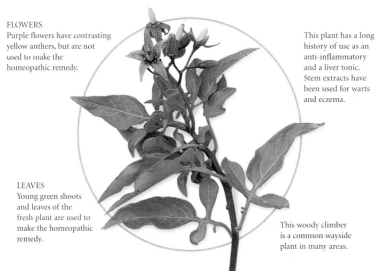

FLOWERS
Purple flowers have contrasting yellow anthers, but are not used to make the homeopathic remedy.

This plant has a long history of use as an anti-inflammatory and a liver tonic. Stem extracts have been used for warts and eczema.

LEAVES
Young green shoots and leaves of the fresh plant are used to make the homeopathic remedy.

This woody climber is a common wayside plant in many areas.

KEY ACTIONS

- RELIEVES PAIN
- EASES INFLAMMATION
- SOOTHES
- EASES CONGESTION

KEY PREPARATIONS

- TINCTURE made from fresh green leaves and stems, which are picked just before the plant flowers. They are finely chopped and macerated in alcohol.

INDICATIONS

● JOINT PAIN
The remedy is typically given to people who are sensitive to cold and damp; it relieves joint pain and stiffness, aggravated by moisture.

● DIARRHEA
Given for diarrhea that may be accompanied by blood. Also prescribed for diarrhea caused by teething in babies.

● SKIN CONDITIONS
Dulcamara is given to promote healing of the skin; the remedy is effective for thickening of the epidermis. It treats eczema, urticaria (hives), warts, and ringworm.

● COUGHS & COLDS
Treats pneumonia, bronchitis, coughs, and colds, as well as associated sore throats, stiffness in the neck, or pain in the back or limbs.

● HAY FEVER & ASTHMA
Eases nasal congestion, constricted breathing, and watery eyes.

● HEAD & FACIAL PAIN
Relieves neuralgic pain, including that caused by Bell's palsy or sinusitis.

● CAUTION
Dulcamara (bittersweet) is highly toxic when taken in non-homeopathic form. The leaves and unripe berries are the most toxic parts.

SPIGELIA

Treats problems of the nervous system ◆ Eases arthritis

Relieves angina and other heart conditions

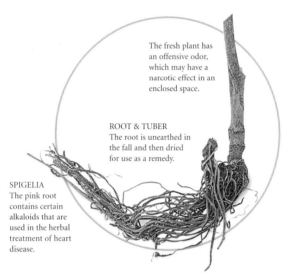

The fresh plant has an offensive odor, which may have a narcotic effect in an enclosed space.

ROOT & TUBER
The root is unearthed in the fall and then dried for use as a remedy.

Grows in North America, South America, and the West Indies.

SPIGELIA
The pink root contains certain alkaloids that are used in the herbal treatment of heart disease.

KEY ACTIONS

- RELIEVES PAIN
- CALMS PALPITATIONS
- TREATS PROBLEMS PRIMARILY ON THE LEFT SIDE OF THE BODY

KEY PREPARATIONS

- TINCTURE made from the dried aerial parts that are macerated in alcohol.

INDICATIONS

● **NERVOUS SYSTEM**
In addition to heart conditions (*see below*), *Spigelia* is given chiefly for problems with the nervous system, especially if symptoms primarily affect the left side of the body and if there are intense, violent pains.

● **PAIN RELIEF**
Given for headaches, migraines, sinus infections, and neuralgic and rheumatic pain.

● **HEART CONDITIONS**
The pink root contains alkaloids used in herbal heart treatments. The remedy is used for problems associated with the heart. *Spigelia* may be given for frequent palpitations that are violent, visible, and audible; for heart murmurs or valve disorders; and for rheumatic heart disease.

● **ANGINA**
Spigelia is also used for angina with constricting chest pains that extend down one or both arms, into the chest, and up to the throat.

● **ARTHRITIS**
Spigelia is prescribed to sufferers of rheumatoid arthritis, to alleviate tearing pains near the joints, which feel as though a knife were scraping along the bones.

ANTIMONIUM CRUD.

Heals skin and nail conditions

Treats digestive problems ◆ Relieves gout

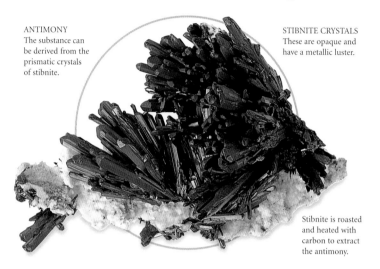

ANTIMONY
The substance can
be derived from the
prismatic crystals
of stibnite.

STIBNITE CRYSTALS
These are opaque and
have a metallic luster.

Stibnite is roasted
and heated with
carbon to extract
the antimony.

KEY ACTIONS

- FIGHTS INFECTION
- EASES INFLAMMATORY
- RELIEVES PAIN
- REDUCES FEVER

KEY PREPARATIONS

- TINCTURE made from
  stibnite that is
  roasted and heated
  with carbon to
  extract the antimony.
  It is then triturated
  with lactose sugar,
  diluted, and
  succussed.

INDICATIONS

● **SKIN INFECTIONS**
A rash on the trunk, arms,
and legs, or itchy rashes
that become worse when
hot, may be treated with
Antimonium crud.

● **DIGESTIVE PROBLEMS**
Given for indigestion with
belching, nausea, and
vomiting of bile, especially
caused by overindulgence
or pregnancy. It is given to
babies who vomit breast
milk and will not suckle,
or to their mothers. It is
also used for diarrhea
and constipation.

● **SKIN & NAILS**
Treats callouses, warts,
and corns that may form
on the hands, under the
fingernails, on the soles of
the feet, and on the tips of
the toes. Also used to treat
nails that split repeatedly.

● **GOUT**
Inflammation and redness
in affected joints is treated
with *Antimonium crud.* It
also alleviates mild fevers
and tense, jumpy muscles.

● **TOOTHACHE**
Relieves persistent, gnaw-
ing toothache, usually
caused by decaying teeth.

NUX VOMICA

Alleviates insomnia ◆ Treats women's health problems

Relieves digestive disorders

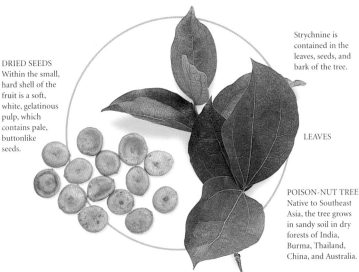

Strychnine is contained in the leaves, seeds, and bark of the tree.

DRIED SEEDS
Within the small, hard shell of the fruit is a soft, white, gelatinous pulp, which contains pale, buttonlike seeds.

LEAVES

POISON-NUT TREE
Native to Southeast Asia, the tree grows in sandy soil in dry forests of India, Burma, Thailand, China, and Australia.

KEY ACTIONS

- RELIEVES CRAMPS
- CALMS IRRITABILITY
- REDUCES FEVER
- TREATS PREMENSTRUAL SYNDROME

KEY PREPARATIONS

- TINCTURE made from the dried, ripe seeds, which are steeped in alcohol for at least five days before being filtered, diluted, and succussed.

INDICATIONS

● **DIGESTIVE PROBLEMS**
Given for indigestion; vomiting with painful retching; diarrhea with abdominal cramps; and nausea with colicky pain.

● **INSOMNIA**
Insomnia with hangover-like symptoms, or disrupted sleep, with great irascibility, is treated with *Nux vomica*.

● **COLDS & INFLUENZA**
Treats symptoms such as rhinitis; dry, tickly coughs; headaches; shivery fever; and sensitive eyes.

● **WOMEN'S HEALTH**
The remedy is given for cystitis with spasmodic pain in the bladder and a frequent desire to urinate; early, irregular, or heavy menstruation; faintness during menstruation; and premenstrual syndrome with a violent temper.

● **PREGNANCY**
Nux vomica may be used during pregnancy to help ease fatigue, frequent urination, numbness in the arms, leg cramps, constipation, and morning sickness.

● **CAUTION**
In non-homeopathic doses, the strychnine present can induce intense spasms of the diaphragm, causing respiration to cease and death by suffocation.

SULFUR

Impotence in men ◆ Soothes painful

skin conditions ◆ Treats gynecological problems

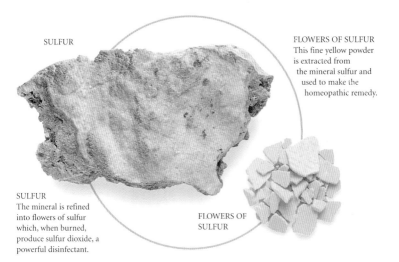

SULFUR

FLOWERS OF SULFUR
This fine yellow powder
is extracted from
the mineral sulfur and
used to make the
homeopathic remedy.

SULFUR
The mineral is refined
into flowers of sulfur
which, when burned,
produce sulfur dioxide, a
powerful disinfectant.

FLOWERS OF
SULFUR

KEY ACTIONS

- KILLS GERMS
- EASES INFLAMMATION
- PROMOTES GOOD
  DIGESTION
- EASES BREATHING
  PROBLEMS

KEY PREPARATIONS

- TINCTURE made from
  chemically purified
  sulfur. It is triturated
  by grinding the
  sulfur into a fine
  powder that is
  soluble in water
  and alcohol.

INDICATIONS

● **VITALITY**
Sulfur is prescribed for a
broader range of ailments
than any other remedy. It
is given to boost vitality
and clear up lingering
illnesses.

● **SKIN CONDITIONS**
Long used in Chinese and
Western medicine for skin
problems. It is used for
diaper rash, cradle cap,
acne, psoriasis, eczema,
ringworm, and scabies.

● **WOMEN'S HEALTH**
Given for painful or
irregular menstruation;
relieves headaches,
irritability, and insomnia
associated with PMS; and
hot flashes, dizziness, and
sweats associated with
menopause. It also treats
yeast and cystitis.

● **MEN'S HEALTH**
Sulfur is prescribed for
impotence or erectile
failure accompanied by
sharp pains in the penis
and itching in the tip of
the penis. Penis or
prostate inflammation
may also be helped.

● **DIGESTIVE PROBLEMS**
The remedy relieves
bloating, belching,
indigestion, flatulence,
vomiting, and diarrhea.

● **BREATHING TROUBLE**
Helps treat coughs and
colds, preventing them
from developing into
bronchitis or pneumonia.

TARENTULA

Calms mood swings ◆ Treats gynecological problems ◆ Treats heart problems

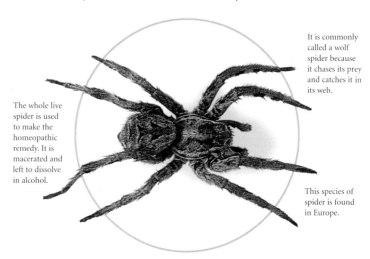

It is commonly called a wolf spider because it chases its prey and catches it in its web.

The whole live spider is used to make the homeopathic remedy. It is macerated and left to dissolve in alcohol.

This species of spider is found in Europe.

KEY ACTIONS

- CALMS SPASMS
- CALMS EMOTIONS
- TREATS CYSTITIS
- RELIEVES ANGINA

KEY PREPARATIONS

- TINCTURE made from the whole, live tarantula (or wolf) spider, macerated in alcohol and left to dissolve. The resulting solution is then succussed and diluted.

INDICATIONS

● RESTLESS LIMBS
Constant trembling and jerking of the hands and legs, usually random and unpredictable, such as that associated with multiple sclerosis, may be helped by this remedy. The spider and the remedy take their names from tarantism, a nervous disorder causing wild, uncontrollable body movements; the disease was popularly thought to be the result of being bitten by a wolf spider.

● HEART CONDITIONS
Tarentula treats angina and other heart disorders, where bodily trembling occurs, and sudden starts or thumping in the heart. Also prescribed for an irregular, infrequent pulse.

● MOOD SWINGS
Rapid mood changes, erratic behavior, or sudden, violent, destructive actions can be calmed with this remedy.

● WOMEN'S HEALTH
Prescribed for sensitive genitalia with severe vulval itching, or where the vagina feels hot, dry, and raw.

● CYSTITIS
Treats the intense burning and stinging on urinating; controls a frequent urge to urinate, as well as possible incontinence when laughing or coughing.

ANTIMONIUM TART.

Heals skin conditions, including chickenpox

Treats exhaustion ◆ Alleviates nausea

Alchemists called this compound "tartar emetic" – it was traditionally prescribed as a powerful emetic.

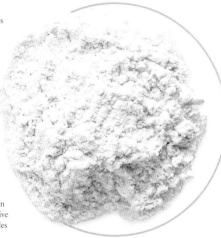

ANTIMONIUM POTASSIUM TARTRATE
This compound is commonly used as an insecticide and fixative to bind dyes to textiles and leather.

ANTIMONIUM POTASSIUM TARTRATE POWDER AND LACTOSE SUGAR

KEY ACTIONS

- REDUCES EXHAUSTION
- RELIEVES PAIN
- EASES BREATHING
- HEALS SKIN AILMENTS

KEY PREPARATIONS

- TINCTURE made by triturating antimony potassium tartrate with lactose sugar and then repeatedly diluting and succussing the mixture.

INDICATIONS

● NAUSEA
Known as the "prince of evacuants," this substance causes severe vomiting and was traditionally taken to expel intestinal worms. The homeopathic remedy treats persistent nausea with trembling, weakness, and fainting.

● HEADACHES
Effective for headaches with pain that feels as if a tight band is constricting the head, possibly with weariness and a longing to close the eyes.

● RESPIRATION
Antimonium tart. is given for severe respiratory infection or chronic bronchitis. Also used to treat whooping cough.

● CHICKENPOX
Treats chickenpox and associated chest and digestive problems. Also heals the scars.

● SKIN CONDITIONS
Antimonium tart. is prescribed for acne and impetigo as well as chickenpox (*see above*). It is also used to treat warts.

● EXHAUSTION
Commonly given for strength-sapping illnesses in the young or elderly.

● CAUTION
Crystals of antimony potassium tartrate are poisonous.

THUJA

Alleviates urogenitary problems ◆ Treats rhinitis
and sinusitis ◆ Heals painful skin conditions

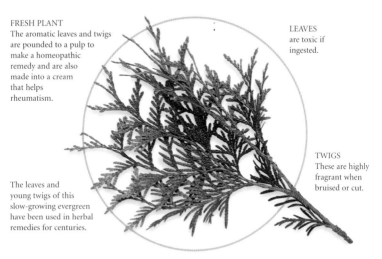

FRESH PLANT
The aromatic leaves and twigs
are pounded to a pulp to
make a homeopathic
remedy and are also
made into a cream
that helps
rheumatism.

LEAVES
are toxic if
ingested.

TWIGS
These are highly
fragrant when
bruised or cut.

The leaves and
young twigs of this
slow-growing evergreen
have been used in herbal
remedies for centuries.

KEY ACTIONS

- RELIEVES PAIN
- EASES INFLAMMATION
- HEALS SKIN PROBLEMS

KEY PREPARATIONS

- TINCTURE made from
  the fresh leaves and
  twigs of the one-
  year-old plant. They
  are chopped finely
  and macerated in
  alcohol, then
  filtered, diluted, and
  succussed.

INDICATIONS

● **HEADACHES**
Treats persistent neuralgic
pain due to exhaustion,
stress, or overexcitement,
or related to inflamed
gums, tooth decay, or
infected sinuses.

● **SKIN CONDITIONS**
Thuja is widely given for
warts. Also this remedy
treats scaly, itchy skin
complaints and brown
"age spots." It is also
prescribed for ridged,
weak, or deformed nails.

● **MENSTRUATION**
Early or scant periods may
be treated with *Thuja*.
Also given for menstrual
pain that is localized in
the left ovary. Ovarian

cysts may also respond to
the remedy.

● **RHINITIS & SINUSITIS**
Given for chronic sinus or
respiratory problems,
usually with rhinitis.
Asthma may also respond
to *Thuja*.

● **URINARY PROBLEMS**
Relieves a swollen,
inflamed urethra, perhaps
with incontinence. Also
cures infection of the
urethra, possibly affecting
the prostate gland.

● **GENITAL DISORDERS**
Prescribed to clear up
genital discharges (in both
men and women), ulcers,
and uterine polyps. Also
treats genital warts,
gonorrhea, and herpes.

GLONOINUM

Alleviates menopausal problems ◆ Promotes good circulation ◆ Relieves hot flashes

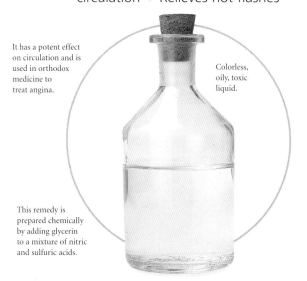

It has a potent effect on circulation and is used in orthodox medicine to treat angina.

Colorless, oily, toxic liquid.

This remedy is prepared chemically by adding glycerin to a mixture of nitric and sulfuric acids.

KEY ACTIONS

- REDUCES BLOOD PRESSURE
- CALMS HOT FLASHES
- TREATS EXHAUSTION
- EASES HEADACHES

KEY PREPARATIONS

- TINCTURE made from nitroglycerine, dissolved in purified water, diluted, and succussed.

INDICATIONS

● **BLOOD PRESSURE**
Glonoinum, also known as nitroglycerin, is prescribed for patients with high blood pressure. This remedy is commonly used to treat the elderly.

● **CIRCULATION**
Symptoms that are treated most effectively with *Glonoinum* focus on the regulation of the circulation between the head and the heart.

● **HOT FLASHES**
This remedy is prescribed when an increase in blood supply causes flashes of heat, similar to those experienced during heatstroke, which surge up to the brain in waves, resulting in severe headaches (*see below*). *Glonoinum* is also given for hot flashes that occur during menopause.

● **HEADACHES**
Homeopaths prescribe *Glonoinum* for headaches where there is typically a bursting "full" sensation in the head; this may be accompanied by great confusion and a compulsion to hold the head and squeeze it.

● **EXHAUSTION**
The remedy is prescribed for heat exhaustion, accompanied by a throbbing, bursting headache, sweaty skin, and a hot face.

URTICA URENS

Soothes burning, painful skin conditions

Treats burns and scalds ◆ Stems nosebleeds

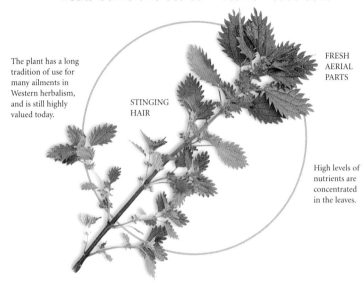

The plant has a long tradition of use for many ailments in Western herbalism, and is still highly valued today.

STINGING HAIR

FRESH AERIAL PARTS

High levels of nutrients are concentrated in the leaves.

KEY ACTIONS

- SOOTHES
- EASES PAINFUL MENSTRUATION
- ALLEVIATES ALLERGIES
- CALMS IRRITATED SKIN

KEY PREPARATIONS

- TINCTURE made from the whole flowering plant, including the root. It is steeped in alcohol.

INDICATIONS

● **URTICARIA**
Appropriately, urticaria – which is also known as nettle rash or hives – is a key condition treated by *Urtica urens*. The remedy relieves the red, burning, stinging skin eruptions that occur with the condition. The eruptions may be swollen or itchy, and symptoms are often aggravated by warmth, bathing, or vigorous exercise. The itching tends to be worse on rising in the morning.

● **SKIN CONDITIONS**
Given for blistering, burning, stinging, red, allergic rashes caused by insect bites, stings, eating shellfish, or contact with certain plants.

● **BURNS & SCALDS**
Urtica urens is given to treat burns or scalds accompanied by classic redness and blistering.

VERATRUM ALBUM

Treats exhaustion ◆ Calms vomiting, nausea,
and diarrhea ◆ Treats for cholera

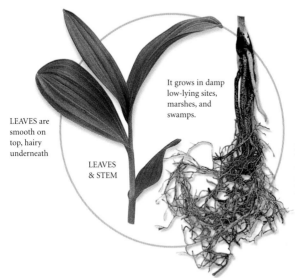

It grows in damp low-lying sites, marshes, and swamps.

LEAVES are smooth on top, hairy underneath

LEAVES & STEM

ROOTSTOCK
The fresh root is unearthed in the fall for use in homeopathic remedies.

KEY ACTIONS

- EASES CRAMP
- TREATS EMOTIONAL TRAUMAS
- HELPS DIGESTIVE DISORDERS

KEY PREPARATIONS

- TINCTURE made from the fresh root, dug up before flowering, chopped, macerated in alcohol, and succussed.

INDICATIONS

● **DIARRHEA**
Along with *Camphor*, *Veratrum alb.* was successfully used to treat victims of the 19th-century cholera epidemic in Europe, helping to make Hahnemann's reputation. The remedy is used today to treat severe diarrhea, possibly with vomiting or painful cramps, due to cholera, dysentery, gastroenteritis, or other digestive disorders.

● **EMOTIONS**
Prescribed for behavioral disorders, such as hyperactivity in children, adult insecurity, or emotional disturbances due to the trauma of childbirth.

● **VOMITING & NAUSEA**
Treats violent vomiting with nausea, clammy sweats, and a cold feeling in the abdomen.

● **COLLAPSE**
For weakness with a clammy, sweaty forehead, blue-tinged skin, dehydration, and possible fainting.

● **CAUTION**
The plant is toxic, although it is said that it is rare for fatality to occur from accidentally eating it because upon ingestion it instantly causes vomiting.

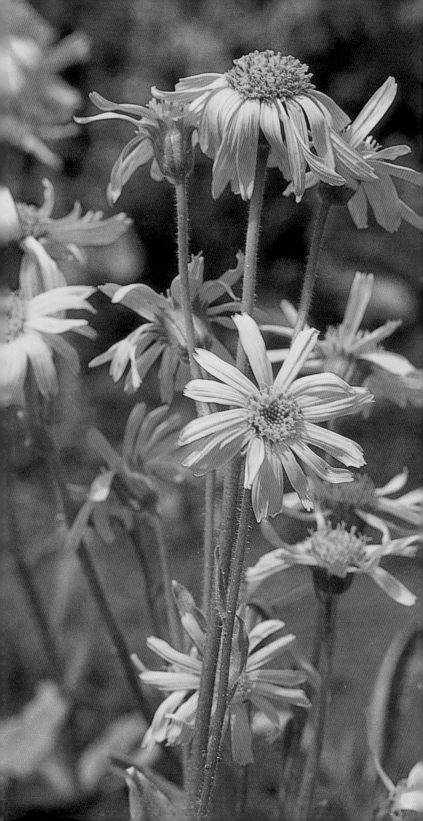

Homeopathic
Self-help

A self-help guide to determining the most

suitable homeopathic remedy for a range of

common complaints so that you can treat the

whole family through all stages of life.

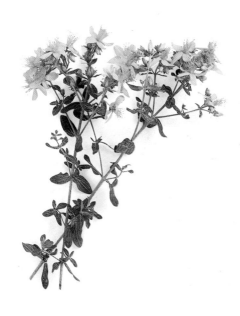

NERVOUS SYSTEM

With the use of homeopathy, the nervous system
can gently heal and recover its natural vitality.

DISORDER	AILMENT	SYMPTOMS
HEADACHE Headaches may indicate a serious ailment, but most are due to stress, fatigue, stimulants, allergy, eye strain, or low blood sugar. Pain results from strain on the head or neck muscles. **Self help:** For pain related to the neck, see a physiotherapist.	That comes on suddenly	•Pain may feel like a tight band •Head may feel full and heavy as though the brain is being pushed out •Possible pulsating or hot, bursting pain •Pain is possibly worse on the left side
	Caused by drinking too much alcohol	•Head feels as if it has been beaten •Dizziness, mental dullness, irritability •Bursting pain in the back of the head •Possible violent, jerking pain or dull, shooting pain in the left side of the brain
MIGRAINE A migraine usually occurs on one side of the head, and is associated with nausea, vomiting, blurred vision, or other visual disturbances such as zigzags, light intolerance, and sometimes tingling or numb arms. Symptoms are caused by the alternate constriction and swelling of the arteries supplying the brain. **Self help:** Avoid stress, learn relaxation techniques, and look into making dietary changes.	Worse on the right side of the head	•Pain in temples and the right side of the head; made worse by concentration •Possible dizziness, apprehension, or anger •Lack of concentration •Memory appears to be failing
	Throbbing, blinding headache	•Preceded by numbness and tingling •Head feels stuffy, possibly with dizziness •Pain over eyes and on top of the head •Rejection of sympathy; desire to be alone •Tendency to dwell on sad memories
	With tearfulness	•Head feels as though it will burst •Pain starts in the right temple •Possible weeping of the right eye •Bruised sensation in the forehead •Tearfulness, timidity, and desire for sympathy
SCIATICA This term describes pain that is transmitted along the sciatic nerve in the leg. It is caused by pressure on the nerve. **Self help:** Swimming may relieve the condition.	Worse in cold, damp weather	•Shooting pain down the right leg •Possible numbness, weakness, muscle contractions, and cramplike pain •Irritability, anguish, or anger
	Relieved by heat and movement	•Tearing pain, numbness, and tingling •Pain extends down the back of the affected leg when passing stools •Cramp in the calf.

The nervous system is a huge and immensely complex structure, with the brain as the control center. Nerve cells are vulnerable to damage, which can range in severity from slight nerve twinges to a stroke. Serious ailments need require immediate conventional treatment, but there is a role for homeopathy's mind-and-body approach, especially during recuperation. The prescribed homeopathic remedies will treat the nervous system by calming the mind, thereby encouraging healing processes as well as by addressing specific symptoms.

IF SYMPTOMS IMPROVE	IF SYMPTOMS WORSEN	REMEDY & DOSAGE
•In fresh air •In warmth •During rest •When perspiring	•In stuffy rooms •In colds and drafts •After a shock or fright •In light or noise	**ACONITE** (see page 31) 30c every 10–15 mins, up to 6 doses
•In warmth •When applying firm pressure •When washing the hair or applying cold compresses to the head	•In cold, dry, windy weather •Between 3 A.M. and 4 A.M. •When taking stimulants •During eating or physical or mental exertion	**NUX VOMICA** (see page 92) 6c every 10–15 mins up to 6 doses
•When wearing loose clothing •During movement •In cool air •With hot food and drinks •At night	•When wearing tight clothing •After overeating •In stuffy rooms •Between 4 A.M. and 8 A.M. and 4 P.M. and 8 P.M.	**LYCOPODIUM** (see page 77) 6c every 15 mins up to 10 doses after first signs
•In fresh air •When applying cold compresses to the head •When fasting •When lying down	•In warmth •During movement •In stuffy rooms •During grief	**NAT. MUR.** (see page 79) 6c every 15 mins up to 10 doses after first signs
•In cold, fresh, open air •During gentle movement •When crying	•In warmth •After eating rich or fatty foods •In the evening •During menstruation	**PULSATILLA** (see page 84) 6c every 15 mins up to 10 doses after first signs
•When applying firm pressure •When bending down •In heat •During gentle movement	•In cold, wet weather •During emotional stress •Lying on the pain-free side •At night	**COLOCYNTHIS** (see page 55) 6c hourly up to 10 doses, or half-hourly if acute
•In heat •With continuous movement •When rubbing affected area •When stretching the limbs	•At rest •On moving for the first time after rest •In cold and damp	**RHUS TOX.** (see page 85) 6c hourly up to 10 doses, or half-hourly if acute

THE EYES

Homeopathic self-help remedies are particularly suitable
for soothing tired, irritated, or infected eyes.

DISORDER	AILMENT	SYMPTOMS
EYE STRAIN Can be caused by overwork or working in poor light. Stress can also cause eye strain. **Self help:** Apply dry, cold compresses to the eyes.	Eyes ache on movement	•Dull, aching pain in the eyes when looking up, down, or sideways •Aversion to sympathy or consolation •Possible symptoms associated with stress, especially after bereavement
	Burning eyes	•Eyes burn and feel strained after a prolonged period of studying or reading •Hot, red eyes; possible headache •Depression, anxiety, critical of others
CONJUNCTIVITIS This results from infection (yellow discharge) or allergy (whites of the eyes are red and gritty). **Self help:** Rest the eyes.	Swollen eyelids with burning discharge	•Eyes water continuously, which irritates skin below; eyelids swollen and burning •Frequent need to blink •Little blisters may form inside eyelids •Bland nasal discharge •Irritability
STYES A stye is a small, pus-filled boil at the base of an eyelash, caused by infection. It may be aggravated by tiredness. **Self help:** Rest the eyes and avoid touching them. Never squeeze a stye.	Inflamed eyes with itchy eyelids	•Eyes are red and swollen •Eyelids itch •Boils on the eyelids develop heads of pus •Depression, self-pity, possible tearfulness
	Inflamed and painful eyes	•Eyes are red, swollen, and painful •Boils on the eyelids develop heads of pus •Feelings of resentment or anger, especially concerning a loved one
WATERING EYES If constant, it may be caused by blocked tear ducts due to infection, or injury to the nose. **Self help:** Massage the sides of the nose.	Watering due to infection of tear duct	•Eyes water due to mild but persistent infection of the tear ducts •Lack of physical and mental stamina •Lack of confidence

The eyes are complex, delicate mechanisms. They are continually bombarded with atmospheric particles, such as spores, bacteria, viruses, chemicals, and air pollutants, which may give rise to irritation and infection. Complaints in the eyes may be exacerbated by fluctuations in temperature, stress, and fatigue, all of which weaken the ability of the body's immune system to fight infection. Although homeopathic remedies will soothe eye problems, standard eye tests are essential for maintaining healthy eyes.

IF SYMPTOMS IMPROVE	IF SYMPTOMS WORSEN	REMEDY & DOSAGE
•In fresh air •When fasting •When applying cold compresses	•In cold, thundery weather •In drafts or hot sun •During physical or mental exertion, or emotional stress	NAT. MUR. (see page 79) 6c 4 times daily up to 7 days
•During movement •In warmth •When gently massaging the eyes	•In cold, damp weather •During rest •When lying down •After drinking alcohol	RUTA (see page 86) 6c 4 times daily up to 7 days
•When the eyes are closed •After dinking coffee	•In the evening •Indoors •In warmth •In light •In warm, windy weather	EUPHRASIA (see page 59) 6c hourly up to 10 doses
•When applying cold compresses to the affected area	•After eating rich, fatty foods •During hormonal changes, such as in puberty or pregnancy	PULSATILLA (see page 84) 6c hourly up to 10 doses
•When resting the eyes •When applying cold compresses to the affected area	•When the eye is touched •During the suppression of emotions, especially following a quarrel	STAPHYSAGRIA (see page 57) 6c hourly up to 10 doses
•In warmth •When applying warm compresses to the eyes •In summer	•In cold air and drafts •In damp conditions •When applying gentle pressure to the eyes •During mental exertion	SILICA (see page 88) 6c 4 times daily up to 7 days

THE EARS

Self-help remedies treat ailments linked to inflammation in the ear, nose, and throat, caused by respiratory infections.

DISORDER	AILMENT	SYMPTOMS
EARACHE This can result from a buildup of ear wax or an infection – such as after a winter or summer cold. **Self help:** Hold a covered hot water bottle against the affected ear. **Caution:** If earache occurs with fever or discharge, see a doctor immediately. Consult a doctor about all earaches in children.	With sharp pain	•Acute, throbbing pain •Extreme sensitivity to touch •Extreme irritability and anger •Emotional oversensitivity
	Throbbing earache with redness	•Bright red ear; throbbing pain •Wide, staring eyes •Restlessness and agitation, possibly with hallucinations or violent outbursts •High fever; dry mouth and throat
	Feeling of pressure behind eardrum	•Pain resulting from pressure behind the eardrum pushing it out slightly •Tearfulness and self-pity •Desire for company •In children, constant desire for cuddles
BLOCKAGE OF THE EUSTACHIAN TUBE This may become blocked by mucus resulting from infection; by swollen adenoids; or after flying. **Self help:** Inhale three drops of lemon juice up each nostril three times daily for five days.	With coughing up of phlegm	•Deafness caused by swelling of the Eustachian tube •Cracking noise in the ear on blowing the nose or swallowing •Runny nose and coughing up of mucus from the back of the throat •Irritability •Anger •Discontentment
TINNITUS Tinnitus is a persistent noise in the ears. It may be due to a foreign body in the ear canal, aging, pressure damage, influenza, constant noise, stress, or taking certain drugs. **Self help:** Two drops of almond oil in each ear once a week.	Buzzing in the ears with dizziness	•Buzzing, especially in the left ear, sometimes accompanied by deafness and dizziness •Deafness accompanied by a severe headache and violent noise in the ears •Possible tenderness in the cervical or dorsal spine and pain in the head •Nervousness •Nominal aphasia (difficulty in naming objects) •Great anguish and fits of anxiety

The ears are intricate sensory organs that provide details to the brain about the body's external experiences, as well as controlling balance. An ear has an outer, a middle, and an inner section, which relay and interpret sound waves. The ears are susceptible to invasion by particles and microorganisms, and are easily damaged, so any pain or other kind of discomfort should be investigated promptly. Homeopathic remedies can be of particular help in treating ailments linked to rhinitis resulting from respiratory infections.

IF SYMPTOMS IMPROVE	IF SYMPTOMS WORSEN	REMEDY & DOSAGE
•In warmth •When applying warm compresses to the head •When the head is warm	•In cold air and drafts •When the ear is touched •When lying on the affected side	**HEPAR SULF.** (see page 65) 6c half-hourly until you see a doctor
•When standing or sitting upright •When applying cold compresses to the forehead	•When the head is chilled •After movement, jarring, noise, light, or pressure •When lying on the right side	**BELLADONNA** (see page 40) 30c half-hourly until you see a doctor
•During gentle movement •In fresh air •In cool, dry conditions	•In hot, stuffy conditions •In the evening •When lying on the left side •With prolonged reading	**PULSATILLA** (see page 84) 6c hourly up to 10 doses
•After drinking cold drinks •When gently rubbing the ear	•In fresh air •In drafts •When lying down at night •In damp conditions	**KALI. MUR.** (see page 72) 6c 4 times daily up to 7 days
•When applying pressure to the ear •When yawning •When bending forward	•At precise, regular intervals •In cold •Between 10 A.M. and 11 A.M. •Following touch •During movement	**CHINA** (see page 52) 6c 3 times daily up to 14 days

RESPIRATORY SYSTEM

By building a strong immune system, homeopathic
remedies help the body to ward off respiratory infections.

DISORDER	AILMENT	SYMPTOMS
HAY FEVER AND ALLERGIC RHINITIS Hay fever may be caused by seasonal irritants such as grass, tree, and flower pollens. Allergic rhinitis refers to those symptoms that occur year round. **Self help:** Avoid all known irritants.	With burning mucus	•Discharge may begin in the left nostril •Pain in the forehead •Possible pain in the larynx •Eyes stream, causing irritability
	In which the eyes are mainly affected	•Swollen, light-sensitive eyes •Burning discharge that irritates the skin beneath, causing mental irritability •Bland mucus that drips down the back of the throat
COUGH & COLDS Colds are caused by viral infections. They are usually self-limiting, but may worsen if neglected. A cough is the body's attempt to expel an irritant from the respiratory tract. **Self help:** Rest and drink plenty of fluids. Eat plenty of fresh vegetables and fruit. Get some fresh air. **Caution:** If there is pain or breathing difficulties, consult a doctor.	Colds that come on slowly	•Mouth feels hot; throat is inflamed •Mild fever; excitability •Nose may bleed
	A cold with irritablity	•Chilliness; headache; sore throat •Nose is runny by day, blocked by night •Watering eyes and sneezing
	Early stages of a cough or cold	•Violent sneezing and thin discharge •Possible blocked nose or cold sores •Desire to be alone; aversion to sympathy
	Irritating cough that comes on suddenly	•Dry, hollow-sounding, croaky cough •Great thirst •Possible rapid rise in temperature •Extreme anxiety
INFLUENZA The influenza virus has many strains. The whole body is usually affected. **Self help:** Rest and drink frequently. Eat fresh fruit and vegetables. **Caution:** If fever persists for four days, see a doctor.	With weakness	•Chills running up and down the spine •Shakiness and trembling; anxiety •Bursting headache, relieved by urinating •Fever; brain feels drowsy; fatigue
	With a high fever	•Fever comes on suddenly •Flushed face; wide, staring eyes •Confusion, delirium, horrible visions •Bright red sore throat

With every breath we take, spores, viruses, bacteria, and microscopic particles of dust, smoke, and chemical pollutants enter the body. The respiratory system is therefore highly susceptible to the effects of atmospheric irritants. Colds, coughs, and influenza strike easily when the immune system is weak, making the body vulnerable. The immune system may be impaired by exposure to cold or windy weather, or weakened by overwork, exhaustion, anxiety, and stress. Homeopathy helps keep the body's natural defenses intact.

IF SYMPTOMS IMPROVE	IF SYMPTOMS WORSEN	REMEDY & DOSAGE
•In cool rooms or fresh air •After bathing •During movement	•In warm rooms •In cold or damp weather •After ingesting warm foods and drinks	ALLIUM CEPA (see page 33) 6c as required up to 10 doses
•When lying down in a darkened room •After drinking coffee	•In warmth •In warm, windy weather •In bright light •Indoors •In the evening	EUPHRASIA (see page 59) 6c as required up to 10 doses
•After cooling the forehead •With gentle exercise •When lying down	•During jarring and touch •In fresh air and sun •Between 4 A.M. and 6 A.M.	FERRUM PHOS. (see page 61) 6c 2 hourly up to 4 doses
•With warmth and sleep •In the evening •With firm pressure to nose	•In dry, cold wind •During emotional stress •After eating spicy food	NUX VOMICA (see page 92) 6c 2 hourly up to 4 doses
•In fresh air •When fasting •When cooling the sinuses	•In cold, thundery weather •During mental exertion •In drafts, sea air, or sun	NAT. MUR. (see page 79) 6c 2 hourly up to 4 doses
•In fresh air •During movement •When warmth	•Exposure to smoke or pollen •In the evening and at night •In cold, hot, or windy weather	ACONITE (see page 31) 30c every 4 hours up to 10 doses
•In fresh air •After urinating •When applying hot compresses to head and neck	•In the sun •In humid conditions •During emotional stress	GELSEMIUM (see page 62) 6c every 2 hours up to 10 doses
•When standing or sitting upright •In warm rooms	•During jarring and movement •In noise, light, and heat •At night •Lying on the right side	BELLADONNA (see page 40) 30c every 2 hours up to 10 doses

CIRCULATORY SYSTEM

Problems caused by poor circulation benefit from
a complete health program that includes homeopathy.

DISORDER	AILMENT	SYMPTOMS
CHILBLAINS Chilblains occur when superficial blood vessels contract excessively because of cold. **Self help:** Keep hands and feet as warm and dry as possible. Apply calendula ointment. Do not scratch. Take regular exercise.	Burning, itchy chilblains	•Skin in affected areas is red, prickly, and swollen •Intolerable itching and burning pain •Great anxiety about health
	Chilblains with swollen veins	•Burning, throbbing pain in affected areas and bluish inflammation •Biting, itching sensation if scratched •Possible tearfulness due to discomfort
CRAMPS Cramps are acute pains that occur when muscles go into spasm. They may occur after prolonged sitting, standing, or lying awkwardly. **Self help:** Stretch the muscles and massage them to increase the blood supply.	Severe cramps in the legs or feet	•Muscle twitching leading to violent muscle spasms •Ankles are painfully heavy •Knees bend involuntarily when walking •Tearfulness and anxiety
	Cramps from muscle fatigue	•Pain resembling bruising •Limbs are heavy and feel as though they have been beaten •Fear of being touched •Oversensitivity to noise
VARICOSE VEINS Varicose veins occur when the veins start to fail and pools of blood build up. They may be hereditary, or result from obesity, pregnancy, or thrombosis. **Self help:** Stand as little as possible and wear support hose. Sit with the feet raised above the hips. **Caution:** If it persists for three weeks, see a doctor.	With a sore, bruised feeling	•Veins are inflamed, possibly with burning feeling, and feel bruised and tender to the touch •Veins may bleed and are sore, swollen, and lumpy •Irritability and anxiety
	Worse for sitting with legs hanging down	•Veins feel full •Chilliness •Veins smart and sting •Timidity and submissiveness •Tearfulness with desire for reassurance

The circulatory system transports blood around the body, supplying body tissues with oxygen and nutrients. In addition to homeopathic self-help remedies for specific ailments, homeopathic treatment according to constitutional type may improve the body's general metabolic function, reduce stress, and maintain the health of other organs. Circulatory disorders benefit most from a complete health program that includes homeopathic treatment as well as a healthy diet, exercise, and a lifestyle that avoids smoking and overwork.

IF SYMPTOMS IMPROVE	IF SYMPTOMS WORSEN	REMEDY & DOSAGE
•During slow movement •When warm in bed	•On exposure to cold and damp •In cold weather •Before thunderstorms	AGARICUS (see page 32) 6c half-hourly up to 6 doses
•With the hands above the head •After gentle exercise •In cold, fresh air	•In heat •In extremes of temperature •In the evening and at night	PULSATILLA (see page 84) 6c half-hourly up to 6 doses
•When applying firm pressure to the affected area •After drinking cold drinks •When perspiring	•During movement •When applying light pressure to the affected area •During sexual intercourse	CUPRUM MET. (see page 56) 6c 4 times daily up to 14 days
•On starting to move •In clear, cold weather •When lying down	•In heat •When applying light pressure to the affected area •During prolonged movement	ARNICA (see page 39) 6c 4 times daily up to 14 days
•When at rest •When lying down quietly •In winter	•After injury •During movement or jarring •When applying pressure to the affected area •In warm, humid weather	HAMAMELIS (see page 64) 30c twice daily up to 7 days
•In cold, fresh air •When applying cold compresses •When standing upright •When lying on the back	•In warmth •In the evening •During pregnancy	PULSATILLA (see page 84) 30c twice daily up to 7 days

THE MOUTH

Most problems can be prevented by good oral hygeine and diet, but minor disorders respond well to self-help remedies.

DISORDER	AILMENT	SYMPTOMS
TOOTHACHE Often an indication of tooth decay, but it may also be a symptom of infection, such as gum disease or an abscess. **Self help:** Rub oil of cloves on the affected tooth and gums, except when taking a homeopathic remedy.	With severe, shooting pain	•Oversensitivity to pain •Jerking, tearing pain that makes sleeping difficult
	With unbearable pain	•Agonizing pain; swollen, red cheeks •Irritability; irascibility
	With throbbing pain	•Gums and cheeks are swollen and painful to the touch •Shoooting pains extending to the ears •Waves of pain that increase in severity
GINGIVITIS The gums bleed and become darker, swollen, and infected. Usually due to poor brushing, but may also be due to stress or other medical conditions. **Caution:** If there is no improvement after three days, see a doctor.	Bleeding gums with halitosis	•Gums are tender, spongy, and bleed easily; teeth may feel loose •Excessive production of saliva •Mental dullness; lack of motivation •Hesitant speech; slow comprehension
	Swollen, bleeding gums with ulcers	•Taste of pus in the mouth •Teeth are very sensitive to heat and cold •Possible mouth ulcers or cold sores •Aversion to sympathy; desire to be alone
HALITOSIS Halitosis, or bad breath, can be caused by tooth decay, smoking, gingivitis, indigestion, tonsillitis, sinusitis, or fasting. **Self help:** Avoid food with a strong odor.	Associated with tooth decay and gingivitis	•Breath and sweat smell offensive •Excessive production of saliva •Tongue is yellow and thickly coated •Aversion to sympathy; desire to be alone
MOUTH ULCERS These are inflamed spots inside the mouth. **Self help:** Avoid spicy, sweet, or acidic foods. **Caution:** If ulcers have not healed in three weeks, seek medicinal help.	Burning mouth ulcers	•Mouth feels dry •Smarting, burning soreness in ulcerated areas •Metallic or bitter taste in the mouth •Tongue is clean, dry, and red •Restlessness and anxiety

Problems with teeth and gums are common in developed countries, where the diet is rich in sugar. Many mouth problems can be prevented by regular dental checkups, good oral hygiene, and a diet that includes fibrous, chewy, non-sugary foods that help to stimulate the production of saliva, which contains infection-fighting white blood cells. Homeopathic treatment for oral infections include soothing mouthwashes for conditions such as gingivitis and mouth ulcers, as well as standard remedies that depend on specfic symptoms.

IF SYMPTOMS IMPROVE	IF SYMPTOMS WORSEN	REMEDY & DOSAGE
•When holding ice-cold water in the mouth •When lying down	•In heat •When eating hot foods •During noise	**COFFEA** (see page 53) 6c 4 times daily for 14 days
•When receiving sympathy •When cooling the area	•At night •When being angry	**CHAMOMILLA** (see page 50) 6c 4 times daily for 14 days
•At rest •When leaning the head against something •When bending backward	•During touch •During jarring •At night •In fresh air	**BELLADONNA** (see page 40) 30c every 5 mins up to 10 doses
•At rest •When warmly dressed •In the morning	•In extremes of temperature •When perspiring at night •During stress •In drafts	**MERC. SOL.** (see page 66) 6c every 4 hours up to 3 days
•In fresh air •When fasting •When rubbing the affected area	•During physical or mental exertion, or emotional stress •In warmth and in hot sun	**NAT. MUR.** (see page 79) 6c every 4 hours up to 3 days
•At rest •When warmly dressed •When rubbing the gums	•In cold and extremes of temperature •When perspiring at night •During stress	**MERC. SOL.** (see page 66) 6c 3 times daily up to 7 days
•When using a warm mouthwash •When applying warm compresses to the face •When lying with the head higher than the body	•When consuming cold foods and drinks •In cold, dry, windy weather •Between midnight and 2.A.M. •During stress •When run down	**ARSEN. ALB.** (see page 28) 6c 4 times daily up to 5 days

DIGESTIVE SYSTEM

Minor ailments such as indigestion lend themselves

to self-help, especially if combined with dietary controls.

DISORDER	AILMENT	SYMPTOMS
INDIGESTION Indigestion is a blanket term for a number of symptoms, including burping, stomachache, and heartburn. **Self help:** Practice some form of relaxation or meditation before you eat. Do not rush your food and relax after eating.	With excessive flatulence	•Digestion seems to have slowed down •Pain when eating even the plainest food •Burning feeling in the stomach
	With painful retching	•Craving for fatty, acidic, or spicy foods and alcohol, which upset the digestion •Heartburn 30 minutes after eating
	With nausea and/or vomiting	•Possible headache around the eyes and feeling of pressure under the breastbone •Tearfulness, depression, and self-pity
HEARTBURN Heartburn is a common form of indigestion consisting of a burning pain in the stomach or esophagus and the chest. **Self help:** Try relaxation or meditation before you eat. Eat calmly and relax for 30 minutes afterward. Avoid eating late and avoid foods that you know upset you. If you smoke, stop.	With desire for ice-cold water	•Burning sensation in the chest •Craving for ice-cold water •Constant hunger
	With craving for sweets	•Laziness and lack of mental energy •Burning sensation from hunger.
	Vomiting and diarrhea together	•Vomiting with burning pain in the abdomen •Diarrhea that causes soreness of the anus and stinging in the rectum •Craving for cool drinks that may be vomited up
GASTROENTERITIS This inflammation of the digestive tract is caused by a virus in contaminated food or water. **Self help:** Rest and drink plenty of fluids (salted, cooled, boiled water). Avoid drinking milk or eating any solid food until the stomach settles. **Caution:** If symptoms persist, see a doctor.	With severe abdominal cramps	•Colicky pains that are better when the body is bent double •Pain relieved by passing gas •Possible diarrhea

A healthy, efficient digestive system is essential for both physical and mental wellbeing, but it can be upset by many factors. Some can be controlled, such as diet and, to a certain extent, emotional stress or allergy, and some cannot, like inherited problems. Homepathic remedies are concerned with improving the condition of the digestive tract, by adjusting the number of beneficial bacteria; reducing irritation caused by some foods; improving waste elimination; and maintaining the organs involved in the digestive process.

IF SYMPTOMS IMPROVE	IF SYMPTOMS WORSEN	REMEDY & DOSAGE
•After burping •In cold, fresh air	•After overeating •After rich, fatty foods •After eating too late	CARBO VEG. (see page 47) 30c every 10–15 mins up to 7 doses
•In warmth •During sleep •When alone	•During touch •After ingesting fatty, acidic, or spicy foods or alcohol	NUX VOMICA (see page 92) 6c every 10–15 mins up to 7 doses
•After gentle exercise •When crying	•After eating rich, fatty foods •During emotional stress •In hot stuffy conditions	PULSATILLA (see page 84) 6c every 10–15 mins up to 7 doses
•After eating cold foods •During sleep •During general massage	•When lying on the back •During stress •After eating warm foods	PHOSPHORUS (see page 82) 6c every 10–15 mins up to 7 doses
•In the open air •With warm drinks	•When bathing •When standing up	SULFUR (see page 93) 6c every 10–15 mins up to 7 doses
•With hot drinks •In warmth	•At the sight and smell of food •Between midnight and 2 A.M. •After drinking cold drinks •After drinking alcohol	ARSEN. ALB. (see page 28) 6c hourly up to 10 doses
•When lying on one side with the knees pulled up to the chest •When warm •After sleeping	•After eating or drinking •In cold, damp weather •At around 4 P.M.	COLOCYNTHIS (see page 55) 6c hourly up to 10 doses

SKIN DISORDERS

Homeopathic practitioners look for the underlying causes of skin problems and the factors that aggravate the skin.

DISORDER	AILMENT	SYMPTOMS
MILD ACNE This includes blackheads and whiteheads. It may be caused by stress, certain drugs, or hormones. **Self help:** Sunlight in moderation and fresh air.	Painful, pus-filled spots	•Yellowheads that are extremely painful to the touch •Irritability and petulance
	Associated with hormonal imbalance	•Spots occur during puberty •Tearfulness and self-pity •Associated with delayed or scanty menstruation in adolescent girls
MILD ECZEMA This is common, especially in children. It may be exacerbated by stress, hormonal changes, or dietary factors. **Self help:** Avoid known irritants. Wear cotton next to the skin.	With restlessness	•Skin is dry and burning, but is aggravated by cold compresses •Restlessness and inability to sit still •Sleeplessness, especially after midnight •Possible anxiety and need for reassurance
	Dry eczema	•Skin is rough, red, and itchy •Possible diarrhea •Craving salty, fatty, spicy, or sweet foods •Anxiety and lack of mental energy
BOILS A boil is a firm swelling (nodule) beneath the skin caused by infection of a hair follicle. They may be associated with illness, being run down, fatigue, or stress. **Self help:** Clean the skin. Never squeeze a boil. Avoid handling food after dealing with boils.	Early stages of formation	•Possible sudden onset of symptoms •Boil is hard and round •Skin around the boil is dry, inflamed, painful, and throbbing •Possible fever, inducing delirium
	Later stages, when pus has formed	•Boil has a head of pus that is on the point of bursting •Boil is sensitive to the slightest touch •Possible extreme bad temper •Desire for no physical or emotional contact
COLD SORES Cold sores are caused by a virus and triggered by being run down or by hot, cold, or windy weather. **Self help:** Avoid eating peanuts, chocolate, seeds, and cereals.	On the lips and around the mouth	•Mouth feels dry •Lips are swollen and burning, with pearllike blisters •Blisters weep before becoming crusty •As blisters dry up, they may develop into deep, painful cracks •Depression; aversion to sympathy; desire to be left alone

The skin accounts for 60 percent of the total body. Homeopathic practitioners tend to regard skin complaints as an outer manifestation of what is going on within the body, and look for underlying causes of skin eruptions. Stress, poor diet, hormonal imbalance, and allergies, as well as infections may all cause outbreaks. Skin conditions may be aggravated by factors such as lack of exercise; eating sugary foods, refined carbohydrates, or other foods; caffeine and alcohol; constipation; the use of cosmetics; and contact irritants in the environment.

IF SYMPTOMS IMPROVE	IF SYMPTOMS WORSEN	REMEDY & DOSAGE
•In heat •In damp weather •After eating	•When the spots are touched, even lightly •In cold	HEPAR SULF. (see page 65) 6c 3 times daily up to 14 days
•When crying •In the open air •When applying cold compresses	•After eating rich, fatty foods •In warm, stuffy rooms •During hormonal changes	PULSATILLA (see page 84) 6c 3 times daily up to 14 days
•In warmth •When applying warm compresses •When walking around	•In cold •Between 12 A.M. and 2 A.M •After physical or mental exertion •After drinking milk	ARSEN. ALB. (see page 28) 6c 4 times daily up to 7 days
•In fresh air •In cold •When perspiring	•After washing •When overheated •Early in the morning	SULFUR (see page 93) 6c 4 times daily up to 7 days
•When applying pressure to the affected area •At night •In warmth	•When applying cold compresses •In drafts •During touch	BELLADONNA (see page 40) 30c hourly up to 10 doses
•In warmth •When applying warm compresses to the affected area •In damp weather	•In cold air and drafts •During even the lightest touch •When lying on the affected area	HEPAR SULF. (see page 65) 6c hourly up to 10 doses
•In fresh air •When fasting	•At around 10 A.M. •In cold, thundery weather •In warmth, hot sun, sea air, or drafts •During noise, music, talking, or jarring •After physical or mental exertion	NAT. MUR. (see page 79) 6c 4 times daily up to 5 days

EMOTIONAL HEALTH

Homeopathic treatments are used to help stimulate a
person's natural ability to cope with emotional problems.

DISORDER	AILMENT	SYMPTOMS
INSOMNIA Insomnia describes a persistent pattern of intermittent sleep that leaves the sufferer feeling tired and unrefreshed. Insomnia can be caused by being unwell, sleeping in a stuffy environment, excess of caffeine or alcohol, overexcitement, stress, food allergy, shock, or anxiety. **Self help:** Increase your amount of exercise. Avoid eating late in the evening. Stop work an hour before bedtime and relax. **Caution:** If there is no improvement within three weeks, consult a doctor.	With inability to relax	•Sudden onset of insomnia •Overactive mind •Sleep occurs eventually but is fitful •Possible painful headache
	With irritability	•Wakefulness between 3 A.M. and 4 A.M. then more settled sleep just before it is time to get up; possible nightmares •Craving for stimulants •Constipation with ineffectual urging
	With great fear	•Nervousness; restlessness; nightmares •Sudden onset of insomnia •Fitful sleep caused by pain •Numbness in the limbs
	With fear of never sleeping again	•Continuous yawning yet inability to sleep •Lump in the throat •Growing apprehension about going to bed; possible nightmares •Rapid changes of mood
IRRITABILITY & ANGER These emotions are often a response to events that are perceived to be physically or psychologically threatening. They can be brought on by overwork, overindulgence, digestive ailments, exhaustion, or impotence in men. They may lead to depression. **Self help:** Increase your amount of exercise. Practice relaxation techniques.	Irritability with over-critical attitude	•Anger that comes on quickly •Awkwardness and intractability •Sensitivity to the cold •Desire for alcohol and fatty or spicy foods •Overcritical of others
	Anger with insecurity	•Craving for sweet foods •Feeling of hunger, but full up after a few bites •Lack of self-confidence

Homeopathy, on its own, is well suited to the treatment of emotional problems. As an holistic form of medicine, it examines all aspects of the individual – physical, intellectual, spiritual – and a practitioner does not separate these elements when prescribing treatment. Homeopathic treatment for emotional problems helps people cope in the short term, but in the long term, it is best combined with dietary changes, regular exercise, relaxation techniques or movement therapies, and stress management in order to maximize the benefits of the treatment.

IF SYMPTOMS IMPROVE	IF SYMPTOMS WORSEN	REMEDY & DOSAGE
•In warmth •When lying down •When sucking ice	•After taking sleeping pills •With strong smells •With noise •In fresh air or the cold	COFFEA (see page 53) 30c hourly before bed for 10 nights
•When lying on either side •When sitting •In warmth •In the evening	•When lying on the back •After overeating, especially spicy foods •In cold, windy weather •With noise	NUX VOMICA (see page 92) 30c hourly before bed for 10 nights
•In fresh air •With warm perspiration	•In warm rooms •On exposure to tobacco smoke •With loud music	ACONITE (see page 31) 30c hourly before bed for 10 nights
•After eating •After urinating •After walking around	•In fresh air •In cold •After drinking coffee or alcohol	IGNATIA (see page 69) 30c hourly before bed for 10 nights
•In warmth •With enough rest •In the evening	•In cold •With noise •After overeating •At around 4 A.M.	NUX VOMICA (see page 92) 6c half-hourly up to 10 doses
•With enough rest •In cool conditions •After hot foods and drinks •After midnight	•In stuffy rooms •When wearing tight clothing •After overeating •Between 4 P.M. and 8 P.M.	LYCOPODIUM (see page 77) 6c half-hourly up to 10 doses

CHILDREN'S HEALTH

Remedies are easily administered to babies and children,

and can help them bounce back to health quickly.

DISORDER	AILMENT	SYMPTOMS
COLIC Believed to be a painful spasm of the intestines. **Self help:** If breast-feeding, try to avoid certain foods.	With crying relieved by warmth	•Bloated abdomen •Distress, restlessness, and irritability •Sudden onset of gripping or shooting pains in the stomach •Pains not relieved by burping
DIAPER RASH The skin may become red and sore due to contact with soiled diapers. **Self help:** Wash the baby's skin with a solution of calendula and hypericum.	Dry rash on sensitive skin	•Skin is dry, red, scaly, and irritated •Desire to scratch as soon as a diaper is removed
	Intensely itchy rash with blisters	•Redness and blisters •Restlessness and a desire to scratch as soon as a diaper is removed
TEMPER TANTRUMS Caused by emotional stress, teething, or allergies. **Self help:** Discipline a child consistently.	Child is impossible to please	•Cheeks may be red if the child is teething; irritability •Possible convulsive symptoms •Oversensitivity to pain •Dislike of being talked to or touched
FEVER This is spread by personal contact. Symptoms subside in two to three weeks, but full recovery may take longer. **Self help:** Rest in bed till acute symptoms abate. **Caution:** See a doctor to confirm diagnosis.	With excessive perspiration	•Throat is dark red, sore, and swollen •Irritability •Saliva burns the throat on swallowing •Tongue is yellow-coated and feels swollen •Bad-smelling breath and perspiration
	With pain on swallowing food and hot drinks	•Tonsils are dark red •Shooting pain up to the ears on swallowing •Restlessness and indifference

Childhood extends from one to twelve years old. During this period the immune system prepares itself for puberty and adulthood. Parents often prefer to treat their children with gentle, natural products to reduce the risk of side effects, resorting to conventional drugs only when a child's immune system is unable to cope with a serious ailment. Following on from childhood, many of the common disorders found in adolescents result from hormonal changes. Homeopathic remedies can help address these bodily imbalances.

IF SYMPTOMS IMPROVE	IF SYMPTOMS WORSEN	REMEDY & DOSAGE
•In warmth •After warm baths •When applying light pressure to the stomach	•In cold air •At night •During touch •When lying on the right side	**MAG. PHOS.** (see page 78) 6c every 5 mins up to 10 doses
•In fresh air •When warm and dry	•When wearing too much clothing or being too warm •When being washed	**SULFUR** (see page 93) 6c 4 times daily up to 5 days
•When changing position •When warm and dry	•When being undressed •When getting wet •In drafts	**RHUS TOX.** (see page 85) 6c 4 times daily up to 5 days
•While being carried •When perspiring •In mild weather	•When teething •At night •After breakfast •While being talked to	**CHAMOMILLA** (see page 50) 30c daily up to 7 days
•At rest •When warmly dressed •In the morning	•In extremes of temperature •When perspiring •At night •When lying on the right side	**MERC. SOL.** (see page 66) 6c every 4 hours up to 10 doses
•At rest •When lying on the stomach •In warmth	•When getting out of bed •When moving •When swallowing •After hot foods and drinks	**PHYTOLACCA** (see page 83) 6c every 4 hours up to 10 doses

SEXUAL HEALTH

Both men and women with problems relating to the
reproductive cycle respond well to homeopathic treatment.

DISORDER	AILMENT	SYMPTOMS
PREMENSTRUAL SYNDROME (PMS) PMS affects about 75 percent of women and includes psychological and physical symptoms. **Self help:** Avoid salty, fatty, or junk foods, sugar, tea, coffee, and alcohol. Exercise daily.	With apathy, irritability, and tearfulness	• Greasy skin, possibly with acne • Craving for salty or sweet foods • Weariness, fits of anger, and screaming • Reduction in sex drive • Sensation as though uterus is falling out
	With swollen, tender breasts	• Fluid retention • Swollen, tender breasts and painful joints • Lack of energy; depression; indifference • Possible vaginal discharge or yeast infection
PAINFUL PERIODS Also known as Dysmenorrhea. Discomfort is common during the first few days of a period. **Self help:** Eat plenty of raw fruits and vegetables. Get plenty of exercise. Lose weight if necessary.	Abdominal pain with depression and self-pity	• Cramp in the uterus causing nausea or vomiting; tenderness in the abdomen • Depression; migraine. desire for comfort • Tearing pain in the abdomen
	Abdominal pain soothed by heat and pressure	• Colicky, spasmodic pain • Irritability, anxiety, fixation about pain • Blood flow includes clots • Dark, stringy, and tarry blood flow • Period starts ahead of schedule
ERECTILE DYSFUNCTION Problems with erection may result from physical causes, or from stress. **Self help:** Try to relax. **Caution:** If symptoms persist, see a doctor.	In anticipation of failure	• Penis remains cold and small • Possible premature ejaculation • High sex drive, but lack of self confidence
	Caused by bruising	• Penis is bruised after an injury • Penis feels sore and tender to the touch • Possible premature ejaculation • Fear of being touched
BALANITIS Swelling and soreness of the foreskin may result from friction or irritation. **Self help:** Keep clean. Use calendula ointment.	With inflamed foreskin and glands	• Inner surface of the foreskin is irritated and inflamed • Possible itching • Possible ulceration • Possible discharge of offensive-smelling pus

There is much anecdotal evidence of homeopathy's success in treating women's complaints. Homeopathic remedies can provide an attractive alternative to conventional treatments such as hormone replacement therapy (HRT) – and are particularly suitable for the treatment of recurring ailments associated with the reproductive cycle. For men, many conditions are easily treated if diagnosed early, and respond well to homeopathy. Neglect, on the other hand, can lead to complications that threaten fertility, sexual function, and even life.

IF SYMPTOMS IMPROVE	IF SYMPTOMS WORSEN	REMEDY & DOSAGE
•When eating •After sleeping •After vigorous exercise •In heat	•In cold •After tobacco use •After mental exertion •In the early morning and early evening	**SEPIA** (see page 87) 30c twice daily up to 3 days, from 1 day before PMS due
•In the morning •When slightly constipated	•In drafts •In cold, damp, and wind •After overexertion •Between 2 A.M. and 3 A.M.	**CALC. CARB.** (see page 44) 30c twice daily up to 3 days, from 1 day before PMS due
•During crying and sympathy •After gentle exercise •In fresh air •With cold drinks	•In heat •In extremes of temperature •After rich, fatty foods •In the evening and at night	**PULSATILLA** (see page 84) 30c hourly up to 10 doses
•In warmth •During hot baths •When applying pressure to the abdomen •When bending double	•In cold air and drafts •After being uncovered •At night •When exhausted •During movement	**MAG. PHOS.** (see page 78) 30c hourly up to 10 doses
•After loosening clothing •With warm drinks •After urinating	•When wearing tight clothing •In very hot rooms •After overeating	**LYCOPODIUM** (see page 77) 30c twice daily up to 5 days
•After bathing in cold water •When adopting a sexual position that avoids pressure on the bruised area	•During touch •After further injury or bruising •After sexual excesses	**ARNICA** (see page 39) 30c twice daily up to 5 days
•In moderate temperatures •At rest •After scratching the affected area •In the morning	•At night •When perspiring •After overheating •In cold air and drafts	**MERC. SOL.** (see page 66) 6c every 4 hours up to 5 days

INDEX

ACKNOWLEDGEMENTS

PUBLISHER'S ACKNOWLEDGMENTS

Dorling Kindersley would like to thank Franziska Marking for picture research, Hilary Bird for compiling the index, and Marshall Baron for proof reading.

PHOTOGRAPHY

The publisher would like to thank the following for their kind permission to reproduce their photographs:

a=above; c=center; b=below; l=left; r=right; t=top
AKG London: 13; Erich Lessing 10, 12.
Geoscience Features: Dr. B. Booth 82.
Magnum: Hiroji Kubota 24bl.
N.H.P.A.: Jany Sauvanet 9, 74.
Science Photo Library: CNRI 18c.
Superstock Ltd.: 25br.
Telegraph Colour Library: Paul Aresu 19b; Ancil Nance 25tr;
Adam Smith Production 18b; Stephen Simpson 19t.

All other photography by Deni Bown, Jonathan Buckley, Martin Cameron, Peter Chadwick, Andy Crawford, Phillip Dowel, Neil Fletcher, Steve Gorton, Anne Hyde, Colin Keates, Dave King, David Murray, Roger Phillips, Howard Rice, Harry Taylor and Matthew Ward.

Text from this book originally appeared in *The Encyclopedia of Homeopathy*, published by Dorling Kindersley Ltd. 2000.